Private complaints and public health

Richard Titmuss on the National Health Service

Edited by Ann Oakley and Jonathan Barker

First published in Great Britain in June 2004 by

The Policy Press
University of Bristol
Fourth Floor, Beacon House
Queen's Road
Bristol BS8 1QU
UK

Tel +44 (0)117 331 4054
Fax +44 (0)117 331 4093
e-mail tpp-info@bristol.ac.uk
www.policypress.org.uk

Part 1, Chapter Two, is reproduced by kind permission of the editor of *The Lancet*

British Library Cataloguing in Publication Data
A catalogue record for this book is available from the British Library

Library of Congress Cataloging-in-Publication Data
A catalog record for this book has been requested

ISBN 1 86134 560 7 paperback

A hardback version of this book is also available.

Cover design by Qube Design Associates, Bristol.
Printed and bound by CPI Group (UK) Ltd, Croydon, CR0 4YY

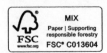

MIX
Paper | Supporting responsible forestry
FSC
www.fsc.org FSC® C013604

Contents

Sources of extracts

Part 3: The sociology of health care

one **Medical behaviour, science and the NHS**
Originally published as 'The National Health Service in England: science and the sociology of medical care', in *Essays on 'The welfare state'* (1958)

two **The hospital and its patients**
Lecture at the Jubilee Conference of the Institute of Hospital Administrators (London, May 1952); originally published in *The hospital* (1952) and later in *Essays on 'The welfare state'* (1958)

three **'Therapeutic' drugs**
Paper given at a conference 'Drugs in our society', Johns Hopkins University, Baltimore, USA (November 1963); originally published in P. Talalay (ed) *Drugs in our society* (1964) and later as 'Sociological and ethnic [sic] aspects of therapeutics', in *Commitment to welfare* (1968)

four **Planning for ageing**
Lecture at the Twelfth National Conference on the Care of the Elderly, Torquay (April 1964); originally published in *Planning for ageing* (National Council of Social Services, 1964) and later in *Commitment to welfare* (1968)

Part 4: Health, values and social policy

one **Choice and the welfare state**
Lecture to the Fabian Society (November 1966), published in Fabian Tract 370 (1967) and in *The philosophy of welfare* (1987)

two **The gift of blood**
Papers published as 'Why give to strangers?' (*The Lancet*, 16 January 1971, pp 123-5) and 'The blood donor' (*Proceedings of the Royal Society of Edinburgh (B), 71 (Supplement) 6,1971/2)*

three **Medical ethics and social change in developing societies**
From *The Lancet* (4 August 1962, pp 209-12)

four **Health and the welfare state**
Lecture at the Hebrew University, Jerusalem (August 1964), revised as 'Goals of today's welfare state', published in J. Kahl (ed) *Comparative perspectives on stratification* (1968)

Notes on editors and contributors

Editors

Ann Oakley is Professor of Sociology and Social Policy, and Director of the Social Science Research Unit at the University of London Institute of Education. She has researched and written widely in the fields of gender, health, methodology and evidence-informed public policy, and currently directs a large programme of health and education research. Ann is Richard Titmuss's daughter and literary executor.

Jonathan Barker directs Far-sight Research, an independent research organisation which explores the views and priorities of service consumers, focusing especially on older people and other minority groups. He directed the Age Concern Research Unit from 1979 to 1986 and headed New York's Accessibility House from 1986 to 1991.

Contributors

John Ashton, Visiting Professor at universities in Liverpool and Manchester, is Regional Director and Regional Medical Officer of Public Health for the North West of England. He has always believed that Richard Titmuss's insights should inform public health policy and health service organisation. He co-edited, with Ann Oakley, a new edition of Titmuss's *The gift relationship* in 1997.

Janet Askham is Professor of Gerontology at King's College, London, and Research Director at the Picker Institute Europe. She is Scientific Adviser to the Department of Health Policy Research Programme on Older People and has published widely in the field of the sociology of ageing.

Raymond Illsley was formerly Director of the Medical Research Council's Medical Sociology Unit and Professor of Medical Sociology in Aberdeen. He has worked on problems of social class and health in Britain since 1951 and was for many years consultant to WHO on health and equity and on health systems research.

Julian Le Grand is the Richard Titmuss Professor of Social Policy at the London School of Economics. He has published extensively in the fields of economics, philosophy and social policy, and has been a senior policy adviser at No 10 Downing Street, and a consultant to HM Treasury, the Department of Health, the World Bank, the World Health Organisation, the OECD and the European Commission.

Michael Wadsworth is Director of the Medical Research Council's National Survey of Health and Development, and Professor of Social and Health Life Course Research in the Department of Epidemiology and Public Health at University College, London. His particular interest is in longitudinal and life history studies.

Introduction

Ann Oakley and Jonathan Barker

Private complaints and public health offers an accessible compendium of the writings on health of one of the 20th century's foremost social policy thinkers: Richard Morris Titmuss. A self-made social theorist, Titmuss was Professor of Social Administration at the London School of Economics (LSE) from 1950 until his premature death in 1973. He wrote widely on subjects across the health, welfare and social service complex. His early work pioneered the subject of social medicine and examined the roles of environmental factors and unequal access to health services in explaining widespread patterns of social inequality. Later, his work on health focused more particularly on the origins, development and success of the National Health Service (NHS) in the UK as a model of public health care and welfare service provision.

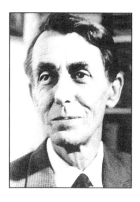

Richard Titmuss

Much of Titmuss's work is out of print. This volume follows an earlier one, *Welfare and wellbeing*, edited by Pete Alcock, Howard Glennerster, Ann Oakley and Adrian Sinfield, published by The Policy Press in 2001. The earlier volume collected together some of Titmuss's main writings on social policy. *Private complaints and public health* performs the same service for his work on health care. Sections of the book bring together his writings on social medicine; the development and organisation of the NHS; the sociology of health care; health, values and social policy; and explanations of the concept of altruism, which Titmuss saw exemplified in the UK's system of voluntary blood donation and which symbolised for him a key difference between public health provision and private market-based approaches to health care. Most of Titmuss's work on health care is less well known today than his later work, which focused more narrowly on welfare and social policy, but it was in the early work that he developed many of his key themes and ideas.

The title of the book is suggested by a sentence from one of Titmuss's early papers on the NHS (reproduced here in Part 3, Chapter One, page 128). In this, he remarks that the advent of the NHS converted private complaints into public ones, making it possible for both doctors and patients to benefit from scientific and technological advances in medicine. An absolutely key theme in Titmuss's approach to the study of health is the tension between science as the basis of what today is called 'evidence-based medicine' and the therapeutic importance of less easily quantifiable aspects of health care, such as people's capacities to care for one another, to exhibit altruism and to form solidary relationships.

We have had three aims in putting these writings together into one collection. The first, noted above, is to make Titmuss's less accessible writings on health available again. Both as a writer on social policy and as a critical analyst of health issues, his work is still widely read and much in demand. Moreover, as several commentators in this volume note, recent developments in health and social policy in the UK and elsewhere give his work a heightened relevance today. Although Titmuss's work is dated in some respects (the last of it was written over 30 years ago), the themes with which it deals are of huge contemporary relevance. These include the benefits and dis-benefits of private and public health care systems; the purposes and values of social policy; the role of 'evidence' in policy decisions; the relationships between 'experts' and 'consumers'; the causes and treatment of social inequalities; the 'problem' (in terms of cost and human tenderness) of technological advance in medicine; the promotion of the health of particular vulnerable groups, including older people; and both personal and social meanings of the term 'health'. Our second aim, linked to the first, is thus to highlight some of the ways in which Titmuss's thinking can enhance current debates about how modern societies can best provide for the health of all their citizens. People outside the UK remain fascinated by the NHS as a health system offering universal coverage. There are fierce debates about the extent to which the NHS is an efficient way of reducing those morbidities and mortalities which are 'amenable' to health care, and whether greater investment in the NHS results in greater efficiency (Nolte and McKee, 2003; Smith, 2003).

Our third aim in gathering together the writings in *Private complaints and public health* has been more serendipitous. Although Titmuss wrote and otherwise disseminated his work widely, he did not put together any sustained, integrative account of his distinctive theoretical and policy perspectives. This is true for his work on welfare – a point noted in *Welfare and wellbeing* – as well as for his work on health, highlighted in this volume by Raymond Illsley in the 'Epilogue'. One can reflect on the reasons for this absence. The pressures of teaching and administration attached to Titmuss's post at the LSE are obvious causes. From the earlier pre-LSE period, there survive various proposals for, and drafts of, books on social medicine. There were also more conceptual social medicine projects that never saw the light of day. These were conceived jointly with Jerry Morris, with whom Titmuss worked at the Medical Research Council-funded Social Medicine Research Unit in the late 1940s. The most ambitious is probably the proposal for a book called *The people's health*, which was intended to "examine the health of the people of Britain in the context of the Society which to so great an extent determines it". There are notes in the archives for seven chapters, including a concluding chapter which would cover "Social medicine in reconstruction and social medicine in politics, in sociology, in medical education".

Titmuss's work in social medicine and health inequalities was, in many ways, a visionary project. It also played a particular role in his intellectual career. Richard Titmuss started out as an "autodidactic, degree-less insurance clerk" (Jefferys, 1997, p 125), working for a large London-based insurance company after having left school at 14 with no formal educational qualifications. It was the experience of his insurance work that schooled him in the mysteries and importance of vital statistics, and that opened the door to a world of 'social statistics' capable of yielding an understanding of systematic differences between the life chances of different social groups. Titmuss stayed in insurance until 1942, working on his statistical and social projects in his spare time, and beginning to publish and become known in academic circles. A connection with the British Eugenics Society helped him on his way to academic recognition, at the same time as providing the Society with a much-needed environmental focus to counter the unfortunate biological determinism of the war years (Oakley, 1991). In 1942, he was recruited to write a volume of the official war history, *Problems of social policy* (see Part 2, Chapter One). Widely acclaimed as an intellectual tour de force, the book secured him the Chair in Social Administration at the LSE, which he held from 1950 until his death in 1973. In 1948, he moved from a position in the Cabinet Office to take a job as Deputy Director of the newly formed Social Medicine Research Unit. Its Director was Jerry Morris, a medically trained epidemiologist, who remained a close friend and colleague throughout Titmuss's life. Jerry Morris, still active at the age of 93 (Watts, 2000), was enthusiastic about contributing to this volume but regretfully had to decline at the last minute on the grounds of having too much to do!

During his years at the LSE, Titmuss reorganised the teaching of social work, established social administration as a scientific discipline and acquired an international reputation as a champion of a social policy based on moral and ethical positions, and as the 'ideologue' of the British welfare state. He also chaired many important committees, acted as an advisor to government (both nationally and internationally), and published a long list of academic papers and seven books. Two of these (*Essays on 'The welfare state'*, 1958, and *Commitment to welfare*, 1968) were collections of lectures and essays. A number were practical assignments. The most important of these was *The cost of the National Health Service in England and Wales* (1956), written with Brian Abel-Smith, which argued that the real cost-effectiveness of the NHS was obscured by the misleading way in which official accounts presented the statistics (see Part 2, Chapter Three). Another of the practical projects was *Social policies and population growth in Mauritius* (1961), with Brian Abel-Smith, assisted by Tony Lynes (see Part 4, Chapter Three). The other post-1950 books reflected Titmuss's interest in income and class inequalities (*Income distribution and social change,* 1962), and altruism in social and health policy (*The gift relationship,* 1970); see Part 4, Chapter Two. During this period, inequalities in health and health care became in many ways subsidiary to his main interest in social service provision. However, the importance of health care, equally and freely available at the time of need, remained the best exemplar of an altruistic social policy, and it was a theme to which he returned in his last book on blood donation.

$$* * * * *$$

The format of *Private complaints and public health* follows that of its earlier companion volume, *Welfare and wellbeing.* Extracts from Titmuss's work are presented in thematic parts, with each part preceded by a commissioned commentary. Although these commentaries differ in style, with varying degrees of attention to polemics and evidence, they all reflect on the significance of Titmuss's work, and make explicit links between the themes in it and issues of concern in the field of health policy since Titmuss wrote, and as these issues have emerged today. This volume also has a 'Prologue' and an 'Epilogue', with slightly different functions. The 'Prologue' is a personal account by Richard Titmuss of his own experiences of NHS treatment as a cancer patient. It was written shortly before his death from lung cancer in 1973, and was first published in the posthumous collection of lectures, *Social policy: An introduction* (1974), edited by Brian Abel-Smith and Kay Titmuss. It is a brief and moving defence of the principle, key to the NHS, of equal access to 'free' treatment on the basis of need. To 21st-century readers, it also highlights some of Titmuss's disappointment at ways the NHS incompletely lived up to his dream of respect for patients and high quality heath care for all. The author of the 'Epilogue' is Raymond Illsley, formerly Director of the Medical Research Council's Medical Society Unit in Aberdeen. Illsley worked in the field of social medicine for many years, including with colleagues of Titmuss in Aberdeen who, in the late 1940s and 1950s, were looking at environmental influences on the health of women and children. In his contribution, Illsley reflects on the historical and contemporary significance of Titmuss's work, concluding that there has been a remarkable degree of consistency in the central themes of the sociology of health and illness over the 60 or so years in which it can be considered to have had some status as a distinct topic.

Part 1 reproduces some of Titmuss's classic early work on social aspects of health and disease. The commentary by Michael Wadsworth highlights the ways in which this work drove forward in new ways, both conceptually and methodologically, the project of social medicine. The first extract is from Titmuss's first published book, *Poverty and population* (1938). This lays out a case for regarding large regional differences in health as a consequence of different social environments. As noted above, much of Titmuss's work on social factors and health was done in collaboration with Jerry Morris at the Social Medicine Research Unit. Their use of vital statistics to study the relationship between disease and the social environment was pioneering work at the time, and an early example of British social medicine, which paved the way for the later development of the sociology of health and illness. In the 1940s and 1950s, social medicine was a radical discipline, the 'social' side of public health. It was then viewed with suspicion by many clinicians and leaders of the medical profession, both for questioning their focus on the individual patient at the expense of a wider public good, and for its perceived ideological bias in favour of public care and policies. These included the encouragement to move GPs to health centres – then seen as an erosion of their independence, now more often regarded as enhancing their prestige and capabilities.

What social medicine provided was a methodology for substantiating the claims of the public health doctors that personal health depends on a healthy environment. Its protagonists in the UK were an eclectic mix of social reformers and/or analysts from different backgrounds who shared an interest in the role of government, the professions and the public in shaping and regulating effective and appropriate services and policies to promote health (Jefferys, 1997). The main strategy of social medicine was establishing statistical links between life hazards, poor environments and poor health. This required careful work in an era when few reliable official statistics were collected and before computers could process large quantities of data and deliver results in a few seconds. Thus, most of Titmuss's and Morris's calculations were done on now yellowing foolscap paper, by hand.

The result was a clear message behind the social class and geographical differences in life chances: poverty kills. Two papers from the Titmuss–Morris collaboration are reproduced here (Part 1, Chapters Two and Three). The paper on juvenile rheumatism plots the social geography of the disease, showing the highest incidence in the rural districts of economically depressed areas. Juvenile rheumatism was the most common serious children's disease at the time; when Jerry Morris started out as a young doctor, hospital wards were full of children with rheumatic heart disease (Watts, 2000). Titmuss and Morris's approach to the "little worked goldmines" (p 35) of the statistics of this disease was to see it as a case study of the relationship between ill-health and unemployment during the 1920s and 1930s. The chapter makes the case for links between poverty and health by arguing for a *dynamic* relationship between social conditions and health indices: health changes as a response to changing economic circumstances. This emphasis on the dynamic nature of the relationship between social factors and health was a critical element in the way social medicine was conceived at the time – at its heart, the subject was the study of the interplay between the health of social groups and social and economic change.

The last chapter in Part 1 discusses the importance of civilian health and disease in times of war. War brings additional exposure to the battle against disease that goes on all the time. But during times of war, civilian and military resistance and the efficient planning of services and allocation of resources are especially crucial, and tend to be more centrally controlled.

Part 2 reproduces some of Titmuss's most important work on the origins, principles and organisation of the NHS in the UK as "a unique experiment in social engineering" (Klein, 1995, p vii). The belief that health services should be provided by the state was a key part of the early social medicine endeavour, both in the UK and elsewhere in Europe (Murphy and Egger, 2002). Significantly, Titmuss himself in these writings refers to 'the Service' or 'the Health Service', rather than to 'the NHS', although his references have been edited to adopt the modern usage of 'NHS'. Titmuss's own interest in 'state medicine' was driven both by his early work on social medicine, and by his research on the development of social policy during the Second World War, when the foundations were laid for a national health service and for parallel changes in social welfare, education and housing policy. These changes can be attributed to several factors: the involvement of the Labour Party in the coalition government; a perceived need to encourage morale through the promise of a clearly different (fairer and more appreciative, if not more egalitarian) society for troops and bombarded civilians to look forward to; the experience of participation (especially by women) in a shared struggle and in the workforce; and the involvement of people like Titmuss in collecting (and, crucially, disseminating) social data and in exploring the implications of these for the nation's health and wellbeing. In examining the conditions of health and illness and the provision of health services during wartime, Titmuss uncovered the soil that gave rise to the flower of the NHS.

The first chapter in Part 2 is from the last part of *Problems of social policy* (1950), in which he summarises the implications for the post-war development of health services of the government's commitment to providing emergency hospital treatment for all during wartime.

Chapters Two and Three in Part 2 link the establishment of the NHS with other policy developments in the field of national insurance and social security, address the question as to why state intervention in the field of medical care made greater advances earlier in England than in any other country in the western world, and consider the impact of the NHS on the experience of health care. Titmuss was very conscious of an international audience here; much of his writing on the NHS was addressed to American audiences, which he felt were often blinded by fears of 'socialised medicine' to the real benefits a non-marketised system of health care could offer. A two-month stay in the USA in 1962 had convinced him that the Americans' misconceptions about the NHS were endemic and widespread (Titmuss, 1963a). From his wartime work, he must have been conscious that this was the most significant element in Roosevelt's New Deal dream never to have been implemented at what was, perhaps, the only stage in American history when such a social contract could have been negotiated, encountering perhaps only the kind of surmountable opposition met by Bevan and a determined post-war British government. The single most important effect of the National Health Service Act of 1946 was to abolish the financial barrier between doctor and patient. Crucial to the Titmuss vision was the view of medical care as a 'social service'. Twinned with this – an equal consequence of the *social* determination of health – was the need for initiatives to prevent ill-health at a social, not simply a personal, level.

In Part 2, Chapter Four, Titmuss examines the impact of the NHS on the standard of medical care provided in general practice. However, he notes, 'family doctors' had to adjust, not only to the NHS, but also to the challenge of a more scientific medicine, the changing balance of physical and mental ill-health, and rising 'consumer' expectations. These parallel developments threatened the traditional basis of authority in general practice; they required doctors to base their treatment on reliable evidence, rather than on individual judgement, and they also propelled them in the direction of treating patients as equal partners in the therapeutic encounter. With hindsight, it must be recognised that these factors also had the potential to trigger increased expense, and they raised new questions about choice and priorities. However, Chapter Five in Part 2 introduces us to another essential Titmuss principle: the inapplicability of neo-classical economic theory to the demand for, and supply of, health care. Here we encounter the Institute of Economic Affairs, a right-wing think-tank, with which Titmuss had a long-running dispute; this helped to sharpen his focus and arguments. It was a battleground that proved particularly fertile for the development of his later ideas about altruism and the example of blood donation (Fontaine, 2002).

Economic issues are at the heart of today's debates about the NHS in the UK. New Labour is committed to a 'mixed economy' of health care in which the profit motive is rapidly becoming an uneasy bedfellow of the principle of public service. The Private Finance

Initiative, the public purchasing of supplementary care from private sources and, especially, the establishment of 'foundation hospitals', reintroduces a potential for conflict between equity and the workings of markets. Everyone in the corridors of power, says John Ashton in his commentary to Part 2, should read Titmuss on the ethics and economics of medical care, and for his wide-ranging insights into the overt and covert benefits conferred by the NHS on personal and public health.

Part 3 of the book looks more closely at the provision and use of health care from an emerging sociological perspective. It focuses on health care both as institution and as relationship – as a complex of needs and services, and demand and supply, in which both the carers and the cared for respond to particular sets of social factors. Chapter One takes up the themes of the social and psychological factors underlying the 'demand' for health care, and the impact of technological development – the growth of 'scientific medicine'. Titmuss expresses the central challenge as the need for medicine to become both more scientific and more social – goals that are not necessarily opposed, but which may be seen as so by some stakeholders. Chapter Two moves the case on to an ethnographic level, recording a critical failure of much health care (however funded) as in a famous phrase, 'discourtesies of silence'. When doctors do not talk to patients and patients are not listened to by doctors, we can see how silence operates: as a device to maintain authority (and define and control demand). The sociological study of patients is neglected, argues Titmuss, anticipating much of the subsequent sociology of health and illness which has expanded just this theme and explained, often with Titmuss's predisposition to improvement in the patient's interest, the relationships between providers, patients and the hierarchies of power existing in professions and large organisations, such as hospitals and the NHS.

Titmuss contributed a paper with the title 'Sociological and ethnic aspects of therapeutics' to a conference on 'Drugs in Our Society' held in the USA in 1963; this forms the basis of Chapter Three in Part 3. (Since 'ethnic' seems a curious word to use in the title we have assumed a typographical error and substituted the word 'ethical'.) The chapter looks at the impact of the 'therapeutic revolution' (more and more drugs for more and more diseases) on the costs of health care, and the relationship between providers and users of health care. An increasingly important group of health care users, even when Titmuss wrote, was older people. In Part 3, Chapter Four, Titmuss considers what kinds of care are needed and used by older people, and the implications of this for the health and welfare complex as a whole. Consequences of 'successful' health provision, both through healthier lifestyles and enhanced care, include greater longevity and a shift in demand for care from younger people (and even young old people) to those who existed only in tiny numbers in the 1940s and 1950s, namely a burgeoning population of people aged 75 and over. This has raised unforeseen issues relating to the social engagement of (and pensions for) active retired people, and also posed challenges relating to the nature and funding of care for large numbers of the very old, whose 'welfare state expectations' are liable to combine with chronic disabilities and a particular concentration of health care demands in the last year or so of life (Barker, 1993).

Titmuss's thinking about health, like all his thinking about social policy, was influenced by a vision of what public services can achieve in a democratic society. An underlying moral agenda relating to equality and collectivism led him to take a particularly broad view of the role of health services. This is the focus of Part 4, the book's final section. Julian Le Grand, currently Richard Titmuss Professor at the LSE, reflects in his commentary to this part on the danger of Titmuss's position being oversimplified. Nonetheless, Titmuss emerges (then and now) as an opponent of market mechanisms in the health care sector on grounds both of morals and efficiency. Significantly, those academics, such as Le Grand, who take a more sympathetic view of the contribution a 'free' market can make to the provision of health care, continue to find in Titmuss's writings a viable and complementary philosophy that demands attention, not least for its moral and public appeal.

Chapter One in Part 4 discusses theories of private social policy and consumer choice within the context of economic growth and increasing social and economic inequalities. It critically examines some of the assumptions commonly made about the operation of the market and shows how market forces are unlikely to deliver either an adequate or comprehensive response to social need, or an enlargement of consumer choice – a point often argued by the economists. Chapter Three is rather different. It reflects Titmuss's interest in the historical development of medical care systems and the problems of population and poverty in 'underdeveloped' countries. It is a brief account of an ambitious consultancy project in Mauritius; Titmuss, along with his colleague Brian Abel-Smith, advised the Mauritian government on social security and health and welfare services in the face of a rapidly increasing population. The two men arrived in Mauritius at the request of the Mauritian government in 1960 in the aftermath of two catastrophic cyclones that had damaged half the houses and most of the sugar crop; they found an island beset by multiple social and economic problems. Perversely, their solutions, which rested on the voluntary restriction of family size through targeted welfare policies, were rejected by the government, but the goals of the Titmuss 'programme' were achieved anyway (Salo, 1982).

Titmuss's last book, *The gift relationship*, is in many ways his best known and most influential work. Part 4, Chapter Two summarises its main themes, using the text of two papers: 'Why give to strangers?', published in the medical journal, *The Lancet*, in 1971, and 'The blood donor', a paper given at a conference in 1972, in which Titmuss reflects on the work that went into *The gift relationship* (Titmuss, 1970). An edited and updated edition of this book was published in 1997 (Oakley and Ashton, 1997). The argument is one about how altruism and social policy can work together in modern societies in ways that are much more likely than market forces to promote people's health. This thesis has had considerable staying power, despite the fact that Titmuss may have been inaccurate in some of his diagnoses of the ills of the US health care system (Starr, 1998).

At the same time, the embourgoisement of British society since the 1950s, combined with better access to information, has raised new questions about the relative nature of health. Knowing more, patients ask more of their doctors and complain more if things do not meet their standards. They also have more sources of information, including advice that can help them choose healthier lifestyles, if they can afford them. Similarly, changing expectations – for example, of privacy or of hotel services in hospital, as well as of new images of 'perfect' health and bodies – have imposed unexpected burdens on an NHS offering free and equal care to all at the point of delivery. One wonders where Titmuss might today consider an appropriate border between public and private provision (that is, when to ask a patient to pay or when to submit to market forces). Communal wards, for example, might have fitted a pattern of living compatible with wartime conditions, but modern holiday hotels and private cars have given rise to expectations about personal space that can make anything other than a private hospital room with bath seem intrusive. Should state care include satellite TV access in hospital or some elective cosmetic procedures at a time when, in England (but not Scotland), the NHS does not currently provide or pay for 'social care' for patients with Alzheimer's who have to live in, and pay for, private nursing home places following the arbitrary abandonment by the NHS of this category of seriously ill person? This causes outrage to people forced to sell their homes to finance their care and met with disapproval from the Royal Commission on Long Term Care (Sutherland Commission, 1999), but it is justified by a New Labour government as an essential cap on 'uncontainable' public spending.

The final chapter is an argument about the interdependence of economic and social growth, and a plea for the ethics of equality to be considered as just as important as productivity in the conventional economic sense. Medical care is seen in the broader public policy context as a key 'redistributive' service along with education, housing and income maintenance. Titmuss's interest in health is accommodated as a central plank of his welfare project, and we are reminded of his unique contribution to social policy, which was to combine the 'quantitative' and the 'qualitative': to link incisive statistical and structural analysis with evidence about the texture of human relationships and the moral values which shape these.

* * * * *

The extracts from Titmuss's writings reproduced in *Private complaints and public health* have been edited to reduce length and too much repetition between chapters, and to increase accessibility to a modern audience. Most of the original footnotes and endnotes have been removed and replaced with Harvard referencing style. Editorial additions appear in square brackets [ ]. References were not Titmuss's *forte* and we have not always been able to track them down. It was his habit to omit page numbers and, in most cases, we have not been able to remedy this. Obsolete terms such as 'the Dominions' and 'the Slump' have mostly been deleted; other terms, which are today politically inappropriate, have been changed; inconsistent references to historical events have been standardised; and masculine pronouns have been pluralised or otherwise avoided where possible. Despite these changes, we have tried to preserve the authentic elements of Titmuss's writing style, and there remain some particular quirks, such as a tendency to refer to writers (for example, Bagehot, Chesterton and Ruskin), without further elaboration.

Dawn Rushen, our editor at The Policy Press, has been as supportive of this endeavour as she was of the first one; we are grateful for her commitment to the task of revitalising Titmuss's writings. As before, this volume would not have been possible without the care and patience of Matthew Hough as copy editor, and the financial support of the Titmuss-Meinhardt Memorial Fund at the LSE.

Prologue: The experience of being a patient

Richard Titmuss

I was sitting on a bench with five other people in the outpatient visiting space of the Radiotherapy Department of the Westminster Hospital in London. We were all booked in by appointment at 10 o'clock daily, week after week, to go into a room called the Theratron Room. I'll explain what that means a bit later on. Next to me on the bench there was a harassed middle-aged woman, married to a postman, who had two children and who lived somewhere near a ghastly part of London called Tooting Broadway. She, like the others, had been brought to the Westminster Hospital by ambulance. She was suffering from cancer of the pelvis.

We talked, as we talked every morning, amongst ourselves and about ourselves and she suddenly said to me, "You know, the doctors say I should rest as much as I can but I really can't do so". I said to her, "Why not?", and she said, "Well, you see I haven't dared tell the neighbours that I've got cancer. They think it's infectious. Anyway, it's not very respectable, is it, to have cancer?". And she then said, "You wouldn't tell your students would you?". By then, of course, she knew me and she knew I came from a strange, peculiar place called the London School of Economics, where she thought a lot of strange, peculiar students had a lovely time at the taxpayers' expense. My answer to her was, "Of course. Of course I would tell them; why shouldn't I use six-letter words? They can use four-letter words. Don't you know cancer is not infectious? And it is respectable. Even professors get cancer". So you see I had to keep a promise I gave her before Christmas.

For many months last year [1972], I had experienced an acute, frustrating and annoying pain in my right shoulder and my right arm. This prevented me from doing a lot of things I wanted to do. And incidentally, it made it difficult for me to concentrate. It began long before the examination period and you know there is one rule that I think students might think about: no professor or any teacher at the university who is suffering from any kind of pain (perhaps stress is a better word) should be allowed to mark examination scripts. Anyway, apart from all that, through my local National Health Service general practitioner and my local hospital, I went through a series of X-rays, tests of various kinds and they all came out with the answer that my trouble was muscular skeletal – something which the doctors in their shorthand called a 'frozen shoulder'. Later I learned that there is considerable doubt about the causes or cures or reasons for 'frozen shoulder', just as there is about a condition known as 'low back pain' among the working classes. However, with this diagnosis, I was fed into the Physiotherapy Department of our local hospital where I did exercises. I underwent very painful treatment of various kinds and, in spite of all this and doing what I was told, the pain got worse and it wouldn't go away.

Eventually, to cut a long story short, I found myself being admitted as an NHS patient at 3 o'clock on Saturday 30 September 1972, as an inpatient at the Westminster Hospital. Admission on a Saturday afternoon seemed to me to be very odd but I did as I was told and I was informed that, if I came in on a Saturday afternoon, a lot of tests and X-rays could be done on me and all would be ready for the arrival of the great men – the consultants – on Monday morning. On the Sunday, the following day, I didn't have any visitors. My wife had had to put up with a lot from me for weeks and months beforehand and so I wouldn't let her come and see me on the Sunday. By about 8 o'clock on the Sunday evening, I decided that I would like to talk to her on the telephone. By then I had learned from the nursing staff that there was such a thing as a mobile telephone which could be dragged round the ward, plugged in and then you could have a private conversation. So I got hold of the mobile telephone and tried to get through. But every time I tried, I found myself on a crossed line with another man talking to somebody else on the same line. After about ten to fifteen minutes, a door opened from a side room near me where I was in the ward, a side room which was used on occasion for amenity patients or private patients. The door opened and out of it came a human being about three feet five inches high in the shape of a question mark. He couldn't raise his head but in a quiet voice he said to me, "Can I help you? You're having trouble with the telephone". So I said, "Yes, I can't get through; I want to talk to my wife". And he said, "But don't you know, there are three telephones on the third floor of this ward with the same number so you are probably talking to a patient at the other end of the corridor who is probably also talking to his wife". Well, that cleared that one up.

The man who came to help me – let's call him Bill – I got to know very well. He was aged 53. In 1939, at the age of 19, he was an apprentice engineer in Portsmouth and he was called up for the army at the outbreak of the war. In 1942 Bill got married. In 1943 he and his wife had a son, their only child. In 1944 Bill was blown up in the desert by Rommel and his back was broken in about six places. Somehow or other in 1944 in a military hospital they put him together again and he eventually came under the responsibility of a war pensioners' hospital attached to the Westminster. Since the NHS came into operation in 1948, Bill has spent varying periods from two to four or five weeks every year at the Westminster Hospital receiving the latest micro developments for the care and rehabilitation of people like Bill. He has never worked.

Bill and I one night worked out roughly what he had cost the NHS since 1948. When he was due for treatment, they sent for him by ambulance from Portsmouth where he lived in a council house and they took him back. The amount was something like £0.25 million. Now Bill was a passionate gardener – that was one of his great interests in life. While I was at the Westminster, a book was published by a friend of mine, Pat Hamilton (Lady Hamilton of the Disabled Living Foundation). This book, called *Gardening for the disabled*, is a great help to seriously disabled people in carrying on a hobby like gardening. Within two days of the book's publication, the mobile voluntary-staffed library at the Westminster Hospital, remembering Bill's interest in gardening, sent up to him the book to read. Bill in his side room was equipped with a small television set. I joined him because, while I was at the Westminster, the Labour Party Conference was being held at Blackpool and I attended it, at least in spirit, most of the time. It wasn't easy to concentrate. A hospital ward between the hours of 8 o'clock in the morning and 6 o'clock in the evening is as busy with traffic as Piccadilly Circus. There is always somebody coming in to do something. There's the mobile shop that turns up twice a day; there is the mobile library that turns up once a day; there are people who come in to take your temperature, the student nurse who brings you the menu card for the next 24 hours and comes to collect it after you've decided between roast beef and chicken vol-au-vent for supper tomorrow; the people who come in to give you clean water; there is the lady from Brixton, homesick for Trinidad, who brings in a very noisy vacuum cleaner. And when I said to her, "Please, take it away, Bill and I are really very clean, we haven't got any dust under the bed and the Common Market debate is going on. It's the Labour Party Conference in Blackpool," she said, "What's the Common Market – never heard of it – I've got my job to do." Eventually I persuaded her to leave us alone in peace to follow the infighting going on in Blackpool.

After the hospital had taken about 18 pictures from various angles of my shoulder and I had gone through a lot of other tests, I was told that what was causing all the trouble was what looked like dry rot in the top of my ribs. So they had to operate. They operated and then they had to have a conference to obtain the right histological classification of cancer. Before the operation and after the operation, I had a seminar (with official permission of course) with the nursing students and I had a seminar with the medical students of one of the consultants. Somehow or other, it had become known in the ward that I had written a book about blood and that I came from this strange place at the London School of Economics where many of my students became social workers. Inevitably, I was asked: What do social workers actually do? What *is* a social administrator? Two days after my operation, I was allowed by the medical staff, by the house officers and the registrars, indeed by the hierarchy in general to go down to the *Paviour's Arms* with some of the old-age pensioners where they had a pint of beer at 7 o'clock in the evening and I had a whisky. I was also allowed to go out to a little restaurant in Ebury Street for dinner with friends and members of the staff of the Social Administration Department. So, you see, hospitals are flexible and this is an area where the middle classes can often get the best out of the social services. I am, I suppose, middle class. I am, I suppose, articulate, whereas many of the patients are not.

After my discharge as an inpatient from the Westminster Hospital, it was rather a moving experience because some of the staff of the Supplementary Benefits Commission had sent me a sort of miniature Rochford rockery and, in a little ceremony in the ward, I handed over the rockery to Bill and the staff were arranging for it to go home with him to Portsmouth. I also handed over copies of my book, *The gift relationship*, to the Nurses' Library and the Medical Students' Library. I think one of the best compliments I was paid as an inpatient was when I was helping two of the student nurses to make my bed one morning. They knew where I came from – they thought I was an authority on matters of this kind – and they said to me, "We've been having an argument in the hostel about the right age to get married. What do you think, Professor? When do you think young people should get married?". Well, I really had no answer. All I could say was, "Not too soon and please not too late".

After my discharge, other cancer patients and I had to attend every day for five to six weeks for radium treatment from a Cobalt 60 theratron machine. Capital expenditure cost was about £0.5 million and there are not many of these machines in London and the South East. I began with an exposure of eight minutes which gradually mounted to about 25 minutes. I can only describe this machine by saying that, as you went into the Theratron Room, you walked past a control panel which looked like what I might imagine might resemble the control panel of the Concorde cockpit. After that, you lie almost naked on a machine on which you are raised and lowered, and this machine beams at you from various angles radium at a cost, so I am told, of about £10 per minute. I had in all about 17 hours. In addition, while one was on the machine, the NHS kindly supplied piped music free of charge in order to help patients relax.

Now, as you will have gathered from what I have said, I was extraordinarily lucky. It was a marvellous ward, staffed by some very interesting people looking after an extraordinarily interesting and diverse cross-section of the British public drawn from south-east London – south-east England in fact. If all wards in all the hospitals all over the country were anywhere near the standard of this ward at the Westminster, we should have very little to complain about in evaluating standards of performance of the NHS. But you know, as well as I know, that not all wards are like the ward that I was in.

When I went in on that Saturday afternoon I took with me John Rawls' book, *A theory of justice* (1973), which I think is one of the most important books published in the field of social philosophy for 25 years. I also took with me an advance copy of the government's Green Paper on Tax Credits, and a bottle of whisky. Anyway, while I was there, I didn't get very far with *A theory of justice*; there wasn't time, there was too much to do, there were too many people to talk to; one had to help – one liked to help – with the tea trolley at 6 o'clock in the morning, when all the mobile patients served the immobile patients, and one shuffled around, not caring what one looked like and learning a great deal about other human beings and their predicaments. But I did read the Green Paper on Tax Credits and, I don't suppose it happens very often, I did write a letter to the Editor of *The Times* from the Westminster Hospital – he didn't know it came from the hospital because I signed it from my home – about the Green Paper because I thought then, indeed I still think, that the proposals, rough as they are, have considerable potentialities for extending some of the benefits of the welfare state from the middle classes downwards to the poor.

In some of the things that I have said and in some of the things that I have written in some of my books, I have talked about what I have called 'social growth'. I believe that my experience at the Westminster provides some of the unquantifiable indicators of social growth. These are indicators that cannot be measured, cannot be quantified, but relate to the texture of the relationships between human beings. These indicators cannot be calculated. They are not, as my friends the economists tell me, counted in all the Blue Books and in all the publications in the Central Statistical Office. For example, nowhere will you find any explanation or any statement about the expenditures by the NHS on my friend Bill and all the other expenditures – public housing, a constant attendance allowance, a daily home help and meals-on-wheels (his wife, aged 52, went blind last year), an invalid chair, special ramps, an adapted lavatory and kitchen, lowered sinks and raised garden beds (provided by the local Parks Department). He was an example, in practice, of what a compassionate society can achieve when a philosophy of social justice and public accountability is translated into 101 detailed acts of imagination and tolerance.

Among all the other experiences I had, another which stands out is that of a young West Indian from Trinidad, aged 25, with cancer of the rectum. His appointment was the same as mine for radium treatment – 10 o'clock every day. Sometimes he went into the Theatron Room first; sometimes I did. What determined waiting was quite simply the vagaries of London traffic – not race, religion, colour or class.

Social medicine and social inequality

Commentary: Michael Wadsworth

The four articles in this part of the volume were written during years of great social turmoil in Britain, caused by the economic Depression of the 1930s, the Second World War (1939-45), and the national experience of structural social mobility brought about by economic change. It is easy to forget now the depth of poverty at that time. In an editorial published on the centenary of Engels' *The condition of the working class in England*, *The Economist* (1944) noted that a study of children evacuated from London had been described by social workers as "dirty and verminous … riddled with scabies and other skin diseases". The same study also showed "… how ignorance and poverty were exploited by all kinds of money-lenders, clothing clubs, insurance touts, quack doctors and vendors of patent medicines". *The Economist* Editorial concluded that "The Government is now pledged to introduce far-reaching reforms in education, health, housing and social insurance, and is planning to bring in family allowances and to regulate wages and conditions of the lowest paid workers".

* * * * *

The contemporary social turmoil and extent of difference between social classes in opportunities for health, nutrition, education and housing caused great concern in both medicine and the social sciences in the 1930s and 1940s. In medicine, there was concern that poverty and malnutrition were widespread and a source of serious damage to health and development (Pemberton, 2003), as contemporary studies showed (McGonigle and Kirby, 1936; Spence, 1960). Social scientists argued for greater equality of opportunity and a more close-knit society (Tawney, 1964), and studied the social effects of economic change (Glass, 1954). Titmuss was one of the social scientists whose work, alone and with medical colleagues, became the basis for the post-war Labour government's radical reforms to increase equality of opportunity, including the introduction of the National Health Service (NHS).

As a result, it was a pivotal time in the development of ideas in epidemiology and in the social sciences. Britain had already an exceptionally long history of epidemiological work. Jerry Morris was a pioneer of the integration and interplay of clinical and population-based epidemiological ideas about the causes and natural history of disease, and of the role of social factors. In the social sciences, the division of academics into theorists and those concerned with social policy had not yet occurred, and the tradition of data collection and data analyses developed by Mayhew, Rowntree and others, continued. The articles reprinted here represent a continuation of the tradition of using what Titmuss calls the 'accumulation of social knowledge' that resides in the systematic collection of national data on health and social circumstances. Titmuss described his contribution as a 'synthesis' of that source material, but from the present perspective it is more than that. Three aspects of his contribution, together with that of Jerry Morris, are exemplified in the articles reprinted here. They are as follows:

- The use of *evidence-based and reasoned argument* as a basis for policy development, rather than rhetoric. In the Foreword to Young and Willmott's *Family and kinship in East London* (1962), Titmuss wrote that "… much of the nonsense that is written on the subject (of the family) today does require challenging… What matters today to a greater extent than in the past is that unfaithful and distorted views about the family do influence public policies". Marwick (1982) commented that, "In the forties, writers and intellectuals could still impress by being portentous and solemn, but in the fifties a more critical appraisal of society had become imperative". Titmuss was, in this respect, well ahead of the field.
- The development of *indicators to delineate social change and change in factors that relate to health*. The papers reprinted here describe social indices of poverty and they have been influential in more recent work on poverty and health, for example by Townsend and Davidson (1982), Wilkinson (1996), Marmot and Wilkinson (1999), Bartley (2004) and others, and in the Acheson (1998) report. The concept of cohort effect, developed here in relation to exposure to the Depression years, was also influential for other social scientists working collaboratively with physicians, such as Illsley and Kincaid (1963) on perinatal mortality.
- The systematic development of what is now known in epidemiology as *ecological level analysis*. This method was later to be used to develop new and influential ideas about biological programming (Barker, 1992, 1998).

In 'Infant mortality' (Part 1, Chapter One), Titmuss uses the national treasure of statistical data to describe the error of apparent complacency in contemporary presentation of evidence about health care for children. He shows the variation in infant mortality rates in the county boroughs of England and Wales in 1935 (the highest was 134 per thousand live births and the lowest was 32), and compares the national rate (57 per thousand live births) with rates of other nations, the best of which was New Zealand (32 per thousand live births).

He notes that it was 30 years since the national rate was equivalent to the current worst rate. Titmuss shows how the distribution of infant mortality rates coincides with rates of unemployment, malnutrition and poverty, and concludes that these are the chief causes.

Titmuss argues forcefully against the contemporary public presentation of information on infant health, giving evidence from the Prime Minister (PM) and the Registrar-General. He quotes the PM's argument that the current national infant mortality rate (59 per thousand live births in 1936) represented an extraordinary reduction from the rate of 156 that prevailed 40 years earlier. The PM ignored both the area differences and the potential for future improvement, as well as the fact that the earlier rate had similarly then been presented solely as an improvement. Even the Registrar-General, who had in 1935 looked forward to reductions in the infant mortality rate, seemed still to accept that a North/South differential would continue. Titmuss wondered why "… it is necessary to wait perhaps twenty years until we can have the courage that reality demands to describe infant mortality today as 'terrible'".

Two other kinds of complacency are brought out in this chapter. First is the idea, referred to in 1936 by the nation's Chief Medical Officer, of an 'irreducible minimum' of infant mortality. The minimum level was thought to be close in the 1940s when the rate for England and Wales was 42.9 per thousand live births (1946), but by 2002 the comparable rate was 5.3 per thousand live births. A second kind of complacency is referred to in Titmuss's quote from a contemporary Minister of Health that "… no one can measure the sum of their [the Health Services'] achievements in preventing impaired health in mothers and initial weaknesses in their babies". That kind of insistence that some things could not be measured was to continue, particularly in terms of such intangibles as happiness, until later social scientists also tried to interpret evidence of ecological variation (Bartley, 2004).

Titmuss also provides glimpses of other important parts of the arguments for new social policy. In 1938, the Chief Medical Officer of Health described the greater loss of infants in earlier times as a terrible "wastage of human lives". 'Wastage of talent' was the term used later to describe the lack of opportunity for further and higher education for all who could benefit, and thus to justify the implementation of the provision in the 1944 Education Act for an examination for entry to secondary education. The second glimpse of argument about new policy can be seen in Titmuss's reference to the falling national fertility rates. He quotes the comment of the Chancellor of the Exchequer in 1935 that there will come a time when "… the countries of the British Empire will be crying out for more citizens of the right breed, and when we in this country shall not be able to supply the demand". Remote and bizarrely expressed as this comment now seems, there was such concern about the effects of falling fertility on the nation's future intellectual capacity that it formed an important part of the remit of the Royal Commission on Population that was set up in 1943. Titmuss and his wife wrote about the "millions of parents revolting against parenthood" (Titmuss and Titmuss, 1942).

Titmuss does not argue here for any particular kind of intervention to improve infant mortality. He does, however, refer to the reduction in the infant mortality rate from 46 to 30 per thousand live births following the introduction in Oslo schools for all children, "rich or poor", of "a breakfast of protective foods". Titmuss may not have known that the low infant mortality rate in New Zealand had been in great part the result of Truby King's intervention programmes in infant feeding (King, 1934).

In terms of what would now be called 'life course epidemiology', Titmuss perceptively comments that areas that have high rates of infant mortality and infant serious illness will give rise to "many premature deaths in later life". Barker's (1992) hypothesis that health and development in early life is the basis for health in adulthood was developed from essentially similar analyses, and inferences from them, using county and county borough data on health and social circumstances.

In 'The social disease of juvenile rheumatism' (Part 1, Chapter Two), juvenile rheumatism is studied using mortality data, with particular reference to children, because of the consequent long-term risk of premature cardiac death. Morris and Titmuss note that clinical explanations for the aetiology of this condition had not been conclusive, and offer the "complementary method of statistical analysis which seemed to us more likely to clarify such medical problems".

Inevitably, they are restricted to the available data, on which they make perceptive comments. They would have preferred to use morbidity data, but note that it will not be available "until periodic health examinations of the whole population are instituted". They note the value of the Registrar-General's introduction of clearly defined regions in the Census of 1931, and also use national statistical data on county boroughs, and urban and rural districts, to show that mortality risk was highest in the poorest areas, however defined. Similarly, they were restricted by the available social indicators, in which unemployment inevitably has a key part, since the period they are concerned with includes the Depression years. They reject the data on unemployment as being "too sensitive to swings of the economic pendulum" and opt for the only other choice, namely Stocks' Index. This, however, is regarded as less than ideal because it is not sensitive to unemployment, being derived from social class of current or last employment.

Their argument is conducted in a way that prefigures comparable work today. The case for a causal role for social risks for the presumptive infectious aetiology of rheumatic disease in children is examined using ecological data. The basic case is made using data on the distribution of mortality by social class and region, and the importance of poverty, whether urban or rural, is teased out. Sensitive regard is paid to the complicating factor of internal migration, the presumed climatic effect is dealt with by comparison with the risk of rheumatic disease in warm dry climates, and the possibility of genetic risk is noted, with the comment in the discussion that "the disease is seen to be so sensitive to social inequality that emphasis on hereditary influences is premature". In concluding that "in social medicine multiple non-specific causation is not unexpected", they implicate "all these factors, damp and crowding, malnutrition and fatigue, lack of sunshine and holidays, inferior medical care, inadequate clothing and leaky boots". In doing so, they anticipate the findings of the Acheson enquiry half a century later (Acheson, 1998). In their comment on these factors playing a part in "the first stage of this long history" (that is, of the natural history of illness), they foresee the life course thinking that later epidemiologists also inferred from ecological analyses (Barker, 1992, 1998).

The paper on rheumatic disease in young people, 'Health and social change: the example of rheumatic heart disease' (Part 2, Chapter Three) moves understanding of the subject on considerably, making significant progress in concept and in method.

Conceptual advance is particularly notable in the idea of interaction of social and disease factors, as compared with the usual static concept. Here three components of 'poverty' are used: the labile measure of unemployment, and the far more static measures of poverty (the proportion of males aged 14 and over in social classes IV and V), and of home crowding. Rheumatic heart disease mortality rates in county boroughs described by these components of poverty are compared during the pre-Depression years (1927-29), the Depression years (1930-35), and the post- Depression, pre-war period (1936-38), for which appropriate statistics exist. Unemployment rose as high as 42% of the insured population (that is, males of working age) in one county borough.

There are three notable methodological innovations. The first is to have examined the association of changing rates of unemployment with rheumatic heart disease mortality after 'correcting' or controlling for poverty and overcrowding, thus making evident the role of unemployment and its variation in rate. The second innovation is to have demonstrated that the association of disease and unemployment was greatest two to four years after the time of maximum unemployment. In other words, as the Depression subsided, mortality 'failed to respond'. The third innovation is to have shown that poverty and over-crowding delayed the 'recovery' of the effect of unemployment on the disease outcome, and to have noted that, after the outbreak of the Second World War, when full employment began, mortality from rheumatic heart disease fell, despite deteriorations in housing. Each of these advances was to be of considerable value in studies of health during the unemployment crisis years of the 1980s (Bartley et al, 1999; Wadsworth, et al, 1999).

It is also innovative to have asked in the discussion how far social services might have acted as 'insulation' against the association of unemployment and deaths from rheumatic heart disease. However, this question is not addressed in this paper.

The publication in 1943 of the short article 'Camp followers of war' (here renamed 'War and disease' in Part 1, Chapter Four) in a mass circulation journal, rather than a learned journal, could at first sight seem like propaganda designed to raise wartime morale. Titmuss questions how it can be that the country's health record is so good after four years of war, when the risk of disease and death among civilians in wartime is high. For example, in the UK, there had been seven civilian deaths to every 10 among the military up to that point in the Second World War. Titmuss attributes the risk to civilians to infrastructure damage through bombing of such vital services as water, sewage disposal and power, and to crowding in shelters, poor housing and poor diet. But, as he lists the reasons why the nation's physical and mental health had not declined catastrophically during the war, it becomes clear that this is a paper about future social and health care policy, and is based on the author's experience as an analyst of the causes of poor health.

The first health protective factor discussed by Titmuss is the redistribution of specialist care services away from the centre, and the list continues with nutritional supplements (including orange juice, milk and cod liver oil for infants and mothers), the new sulphonamide class of drugs, improved medical care and diagnosis, and full employment and regular wages. With the exception of the distribution of specialist services, these protective factors are the obverse of the health risks identified by Titmuss and Morris in their earlier papers on health topics. They had shown the profound health risks associated with poverty, and described their uneven social and geographical distribution.

We may be sure that this article is about future national health care policy because of its timing, content, and publication in *The Listener*. Publication of this article coincides with the period of discussion about post-war transformation of health, education and welfare services, and when arguments for and against a national health service were being discussed. The redistribution and increase of specialist health services was clearly going to be necessary for a national health service, as were national policies to maintain employment and earnings, as well as adequate nutrition. Publication in *The Listener*, which was widely read among the classes concerned with opinion formation and policy development, as well as among politicians and voters, may be interpreted as a shrewd use of new knowledge gained through research published in respected, peer-reviewed journals. Such awareness of political expediency and such follow-through from research to policy development was a hallmark of the Titmuss style, and of the social medicine of the period.

Infant mortality

It was, I think, Sir Josiah Stamp who stressed the need for mobilising the facts of modern society that scientific research has brought to light.

A fact, per se, is of little value unless it be, first, disposed in its proper context; second, related to allied established facts and knowledge; and third, understood and interpreted in terms of its influence and importance on other facts and on the whole field of social knowledge. When that point is reached, understanding must be translated into action. The measured facts of human birth, life and death, expressed in terms of the pain and suffering that is past, must be used to transform the conditions of the living.

The aggregate of accumulated social knowledge is now so diverse, so vast, that as a result of enforced specialisation, each branch of scientific research tends to be driven into isolation. Unfortunately, for many research workers isolation spells academic meaninglessness. Therefore, despite the great advance in knowledge, we may still retain a nodding acquaintance with the attitude which resulted in the British Navy taking 200 years to realise that scurvy was caused by inadequate diet.

It is to be deplored that so much valuable information, so many relevant facts, are lost and buried in the avalanche of statistics, blue books, reports, bulletins, books and research pamphlets that descend on the sociologist every year. In my book, *Poverty and population* (1938), I have rescued a few of these facts from threatened eclipse.

On a personal note, I recognise that it is my wife, Kay – not only by her part in the publication of this book, but through her work among the unemployed and forgotten men and women of London – who has helped me to visualise the human significance, and often the human tragedy, hidden behind each fact, and the social waste that the forces of poverty and unemployment relentlessly generate.

* * * * *

The Prime Minister, Ramsey MacDonald, speaking at Edinburgh on 12 November 1937, said, in discussing public health, "sometimes we take infant mortality rates as a sort of general pointer to show how health is improving. If you do that, the story is very wonderful, because in the last 40 years … that is not much more than half my own lifetime … the infant mortality rate has come down from 156 to 59 per 1,000".

Enlarging on the subject of this improvement, Sir Arthur MacNalty, the Chief Medical Officer of Health, in his Introduction to the Annual Report (1936), states:

> Maternity and child welfare continues to hold a prominent place in public interest both in this and in other countries. There is a real concern that unnecessary suffering and illness of both mothers and children should be avoided and that the toll of deaths should be reduced as far as this is humanly possible. There is a universal desire that maternity should be safeguarded and that young children should be given every opportunity for development which makes for healthy growth and for well-being in both body and mind.

In his report, MacNalty illustrates the saving of life by saying, "In 1936, 35,425 infants died under one year of age. If the 1901-10 rate had obtained in 1936, 77,477 infants would have died in the latter year. There has, therefore, been a saving to the country of about 42,000 lives of the newly-born". Later he notes that, "Nothing is more remarkable than the decrease in infant mortality in the last 30 years, and, as was noted in the Annual Report for 1933, no spectacular improvement can now be anticipated. The lower the rate, the nearer one approaches the irreducible minimum". By adopting, however, the same approach as the Chief Medical Officer, it appears that if the same conditions and the same infant mortality rates that existed in 1936 in many towns of a 'depressed' nature, such as Jarrow and Gelligaer (South Wales), had obtained throughout the whole of England and Wales, the nation would have lost in that one year approximately 25,000 more infants.

Yet similarly high rates operative in the quinquennium 1896-1900 were stigmatised by the Chief Medical Officer of Health (*Daily Telegraph and Morning Post Fitness Supplement*, 17 January 1938) as "the wastage of human lives in the process [of improvement] has been terrible in the past". When in this country in 10 to 20 years' time the day-to-day state of the birth rate may well be 'front page news', it is difficult to avoid the conclusion that the wastage today may equally be described as 'terrible'. Judged from the quantitative aspects and ignoring any humanitarian standards, the attitude of complacency in 1901 based on improvement over the preceding 40 years was perhaps understandable, but today [1938], equipped with the great advances that medical knowledge has made and in the light of an impending population decline, but while still oblivious to the sum total of human pain, can it be justified? Why, then, is it necessary to wait perhaps 20 years until we can have the courage that reality demands to describe infant mortality today as 'terrible'? Despite, therefore, the opinion of the Chief Medical Officer of Health, it is not apparent from a thorough analysis of the geographical distribution of infant mortality that we are yet approaching the 'irreducible minimum'.

It is inconceivable that there can be more than one 'irreducible minimum' in the world, yet New Zealand has reduced infant mortality to 32 per 1,000 live births (1935) as against 57 for England and Wales (1935) and 59 (1936). (See Table 1.)

The fact that there are many countries in Europe and the rest of the world with a higher infant mortality rate is irrelevant while such wide divergencies exist within England and Wales.

Assuming that England and Wales as a whole achieve a national death rate equivalent to that prevailing in New Zealand, we should save over 16,000 infants per annum out of a total number of 35,425 deaths. Unless and until, however, those factors obtaining in the South (and in New Zealand, Scandinavia, and so on), conducive to a decline in infant mortality, prevail *pari passu* in the North and Wales, we can look for no 'spectacular improvement'. But, as this improved rate has been achieved in some parts of the country, there appears to be no fundamental reason why it should not also obtain throughout England and Wales. That there is ground for improvement is exemplified by the tabulated statistics which disclose that over 5,000 excess deaths occurred among infants under the age of one in the North and Wales during 1936, or something like 30,000 surplus deaths since the slump of 1931.

The standard for measuring public health is surely not what was but what might be. As long as we fall short of that standard, there is scope for improvement.

Table 1: Infant mortality: comparisons with other countries, 1935 (per 1,000 live births)

Coulsdon and Purley	32	New Zealand	32
Surrey	41	Natal	32
Home Counties	42	South Australia	35
South East as a whole	47	Queensland	37
Middlesex	48	New South Wales	39
Greater London	51	Australia as a whole	40
Midlands	59	Holland	40
Wales	63	Sweden	47
Glamorgan	63	Norway	48
North*	68	Switzerland	48
Gelligaer	74	Province of Ontario (comprising one third of	56
North I*	76	total population of Canada)	
Durham	76	US	60
Scotland	77	Union of South Africa	64
Sunderland	92	Germany	68
Jarrow M.B.	114	Canada as a whole	71
Riverside Area, Stockton-on Tees, mean of 1928-32	134		

*This is how the data appeared in the original version; the difference between 'North' and 'North I' is not known.

For example, one has to go back 21 years to find an infant mortality rate for England and Wales that exceeds that for Jarrow in 1936.

If one compares Jarrow with a community in the South East of roughly the same size, for example Coulsdon and Purley, the results disclose an excess of infant mortality of 222%. Gelligaer, an urban district (like Coulsdon and Purley) in South Wales and approximately the same size, has an excess of 157%.

In the realisation of what all this social waste involves, the words of Sir Kingsley Wood on 5 October 1927, when Parliamentary Secretary to the Ministry of Health, that the infant death rate is "one of the best tests of health progress" should not be forgotten.

The evidence shows that out of 401 deaths in Durham from bronchitis, pneumonia and other respiratory diseases, two thirds (or 266) would not have occurred if the conditions in Surrey had prevailed in Durham. This hardly constitutes an endorsement of the Minister of Health's statement, when praising our health services, that "no one can measure the sum of their achievements in preventing impaired health in mothers and initial weaknesses in their babies, and in setting the latter firmly on their upward path. For these services are not just saving lives – they are making better the lives that are saved as well".

An analysis of neo-natal deaths at different ages (for example, 1, 2, 3, 4, 5 and 6 days, and 1 to 4 weeks) exhibits similar upward trends from the South to Wales and the North; likewise, infant mortality at ages over one month to one year.

A comparison of the distribution of infant mortality from some of the principal causes in 1935 is also indicative (Table 2).

The excessive mortality from measles and whooping cough implies a widespread prevalence of rickets, because a reduction in these two diseases has been ascribed to a diminished incidence of rickets. Further, a decline in rickets has been paralleled by a reduction in the prevalence of epidemic diarrhoea. This disease, with its terrible drain on nutrition and the occurrence of prolonged 'marasmus'[1] is far more widespread in the North and Wales than in the South East, and thereby leaves

Table 2: Infant mortality from some of the principal causes by region (rates per 100 of those for England and Wales)

	Measles	Whooping cough	Tuberculosis (all forms)	Bronchitis and pneumonia	Congenital debility	Convulsions
England and Wales	100	100	100	100	100	100
'Standard'	17	61	93	58	80	48
North*	188	129	98	132	135	147
North I*	217	163	121	142	163	222
Wales*	154	113	105	111	124	248
Wales I*	208	121	91	117	137	241

*This is how the data appeared in the original version; the difference between 'North' and 'North I', and 'Wales' and 'Wales I' are not known.

behind many debilitated, rachitic survivors. The relatively high incidence, therefore, in the North and Wales, of these crippling diseases not only implies malnutrition and poverty but also accounts for many premature deaths later in life. T.H.C. Stevenson showed in the Registrar-General's Annual Report, 1911, that diarrhoeal mortality was far heavier among the poor than the well-to-do.

The Registrar-General (1935 Review), in analysing the causes of high infant mortality in certain county boroughs, states in connection with congenital malformations and diseases of early infancy (accountable for the majority of deaths under one year of age) that "large numbers of these deaths are due to remediable causes and that considerable improvement in the death rate from this group of causes is possible of achievement in many large towns". He concludes by stating that "it ought to be possible for every northern town to achieve a rate below 50 (infant mortality) and for every other town to achieve a rate below 40. The realisation of such rates would mean an annual saving of more than 4,000 infant lives in the County Boroughs alone". Apart from suggesting that, because divergencies have existed in the past, they should continue to do so in the future, it is difficult to justify the distinction in the risk of infant survival between the North and other parts of the country.

Assuming, however, the realisation (apparently 'practical politics') of a rate of, say 45 per 1,000 live births for the whole of England and Wales, this would effect an annual saving in infant life of over 8,000, or by 1946 of something like 60,000 to 70,000 future citizens. On the practicability of achieving improvement, it is of interest to note the results of the Oslo experiment. Every child in the town, rich or poor, can have at school a breakfast of protective foods which brings their diet up to a higher standard. This, together with other measures for improving housing and feeding, has raised the national level of health considerably. The infant mortality rate in Oslo, which was 46 in 1931, is now [1938] down to 30.

So far as the North of England and Wales is concerned, there appears little doubt, by studying area by area the rise and fall of infant mortality with the incidence of unemployment, overcrowding, public assistance and trade depression, that these unnecessary deaths are caused in the main by malnutrition in the mother and/or child, or, in other words, poverty.

To emphasise the fundamental importance of the interaction of infant mortality on the problems surrounding the future of the population, it is as well to quote again the words of the Prime Minister, Ramsey MacDonald. He said, when delivering his Budget Speech as Chancellor of the Exchequer on 15 April 1935:

> I must say that I look upon the continued diminution of
> the birth rate in this country with considerable apprehension.

At the present time, it may seem that we have here a larger population than we are able to support in England. At the same time, we know the difficulties which the Dominions find in accommodating a larger population, when they themselves are troubled with unemployment. But I have a feeling that the time may not be far distant when that position will be reversed, when the countries of the British Empire will be crying out for more citizens of the right breed, and when we in this country shall not be able to supply the demand.

From a study of the differential regional birth rates, it is abundantly clear that it is only the higher fertility rates in the North and Wales which are saving the country from a more rapid, and consequently more disastrous, decline in population. If the birth rate (live births per 1,000 women aged 15 to 44) which obtained in the whole of the South East of England in 1936 had also applied to the North and Wales, there would have been over 25,000 fewer births. If this rate in the South East had obtained throughout the whole of England and Wales, the number of future potential parents would have been reduced in one year by over 40,000. Obversely, if the birth rate for Durham and Northumberland in 1936 had operated in the South East in the same year, we should have had over 55,000 more children (an increase of 29% for the latter area), and if for the whole of England and Wales, over 115,000 more (an increase of 21%). These are, of course, only approximate figures, but, after allowing even a considerable margin of error, they still indicate the basic nature and extent of the problems and impress, not only by the range of the figures, but by the social implications which underlie them.

Our child population is steadily declining. If the children born today are, as an integral part of our population, our chief national asset – "There is no wealth but life ... that country is the richest which nourishes the greatest number of noble and happy human beings" (Ruskin) – then it hardly seems an ideal arrangement to allow the major proportion of those children who survive the 'terrible wastage' to grow to manhood and womanhood in those areas known to be most depressed and most exposed to malnutrition. Neither, let it be said, can we, in face of the uneven risks attending entry into life, lay claim to 'the democracy of birth' in this country.

Note

[1] The term marasmus, now obsolete, was commonly used in medical texts around the 1940s and is defined as 'the condition in a child of having a weight less than 60% of the normal for his or her age' (*Oxford English Dictionary*).

The social disease of juvenile rheumatism

Juvenile rheumatism is the least known of the great infectious diseases. The cause is obscure, the diagnosis often doubtful and the treatment symptomatic. Incidence and mortality are equally uncertain. The peculiar natural history of the disease and the lack of adequate statistics make the incidence difficult to estimate. For knowledge of the mortality, we are largely dependent on the Registrar-General's reports, and they are not directly concerned with rheumatism as a cause of heart disease. The immediate infective agent of the disease is still undefined but much information has accumulated on the predisposing factors. In America, hereditary influences are increasingly stressed; in the UK, the malady has long been recognised as one of the group of social diseases.

* * * * *

Several attempts have been made to measure the prevalence of the infection.

The Ministry of Health report on acute rheumatism (1927) estimated that 2% of the elementary-school population "in cities and towns require observation … on account of manifestations of rheumatic infection". Among insured adults, a previous investigation (1924) found that the annual attack-rate for acute and subacute rheumatism was approximately 4.5 per 1,000 and that 2.5% of all sickness absence was due to rheumatic conditions. Davidson and Duthie (1938), on the basis of a large sample study, suggested that the annual rate for the whole population of Scotland was 6.5 per 1,000. The disease seems to be declining in severity and commonness (Close, 1930; Miller, 1937), although Thornton (1938) estimated that in the London County Council area the incidence in elementary-school children was still 2.5%.

Mortality from rheumatic fever has been falling with temporary interruptions for many years. In 1881-90 the rate per million living at all ages was 95, in 1911-20 it was 50, and in 1939 it was 25. But rheumatic fever is important only in childhood. The trend here has not been so satisfactory. At 5-10 and 10-15 years, mortality in 1881-90 was 67 and 103; in 1911-20 the corresponding rates were 62 and 86; and in 1936-38 they were 50 and 60.

* * * * *

Clinical experience must determine the rheumatic proportion of deaths from rheumatic heart disease, and various series of cases (Wyckoff and Ling, 1926; Grant, 1933) are available which indicate the age distribution of the different ætiological types. Of Grant's 1,000 ex-soldiers with heart disease, the rheumatic group was approximately 80% of the total in their twenties, 65% in their thirties, 28% in their forties and 18% in their fifties. In Wyckoff and Ling's series of New York clinics and private patients, about 9% of the cases between 50 and 59 years and 4% of those over 60 years were rheumatic. Such percentages could be considered, by analogy, the rheumatic fraction of all cardiac deaths in the decade specified, although there are obvious sources of error in such a method. A check is provided by information on the expectation of life in patients with rheumatic heart disease. In De Graff and Ling's adult cases (1935), the average age of death was 33; of Coomb's (1924) English series, only 7% reached the age of 50. Hedley (1940), in a large-scale investigation, found that more than 50% of the deaths occurred under 30 years and only 3% over 60. In New York (Swift, 1940), where practitioners are now [1942] requested to specify rheumatism when applicable in deaths from heart disease, 40% of the cases so reported in 1938 were under 30, 44% between 30 and 60.

In view of the nature of such data, any estimate of mortality from rheumatic heart disease is bound to be rather speculative. The clinical evidence available suggests that the mortality was near 10,000 in 1938 and 11,000 in 1930. Since the total number of deaths from heart disease under 45 in these years was 6,722 and 7,434, the current concept of the age incidence of juvenile rheumatism must be erroneous if the higher estimates of 25,000 and 30,000 are more correct.

Rheumatism now causes about 10% of all deaths from heart disease, and close on 100% of those occurring under the age of 40. Combining rheumatic fever, chorea and rheumatic heart disease, juvenile rheumatism is responsible for approximately 2% of all deaths in England and Wales, and for 10% between 5 and 45, when it is second only in females to phthisis, and follows phthisis.[1]

The total estimates just reached are so hypothetical that to judge mortality trends from a series of such would be pointless. Instead, we have used all diseases of the circulatory system at 5 to 25 – a crude but adequate index. Mortality during the 1920s was at a considerably lower level than in the period up to 1918. In adolescents and young adults, the second retardation in the 1920s and 1930s is rather reminiscent of recent experience in phthisis. Since 1937, there has been a general improvement.

Routine school inspection (Chief Medical Officer, 1940) has shown that just over five children per 1,000 or fewer than 30,000 in all, have organic heart disease. In London, Thornton (1938) reported the incidence as 2% in 1926 and 0.8% in 1936. In adults, it is impossible to state the incidence with any accuracy. Among insured workers, the report on incapacitating sickness showed that, under the age of 35, the number of new cases of heart disease per annum was about two per 1,000 in men, just under three in single women, and just over three in married women. In these groups, the number ill of heart disease over the whole year was 0.12 per 1,000, 0.35 and 0.41. Berkeley et al (1938) indicate that 1-2.5% of all pregnant women have rheumatic heart disease. Periodic health examinations are rare in this country; Morris (1941) found the incidence to be 1% in a sample of 1,352 adult males. Another source of information is De Graff and Ling's (1935) series where 15 years was the average between onset of the disease and final heart failure. On the number of adult deaths already estimated, there appear to be 125,000-150,000 cases in England and Wales. Paul (1943) considered the incidence to be approximately 8.4 per 1,000.

It can be hazarded that there are nearly 200,000 cases of rheumatic heart disease at all ages in the UK. This probably gives juvenile rheumatism the melancholy distinction of being first among all infections as a cause of chronic illness and disablement; chronic, but punctuated with frequent acuter episodes and occurring almost entirely in what should be the most useful years of life.

* * * * *

Juvenile rheumatism may be 30 times more prevalent among the poor than the well-to-do (Glover, 1930). The British Medical Association Committee (Miller, 1926), however, agreed with some earlier authorities and suggested that the incidence was more selective, being higher in the artisan class than among the very poor. This is an observation of great interest and has been variously explained by Miller (1934b), Wilkinson (1935) and Poynton (1938). It has also been disputed by Hill (1930), Glover (1934) and in the reports of the Kensington Rheumatism Scheme.

In the Occupational Mortality Supplements, those little worked goldmines, the Registrar-General classifies deaths according to the occupational (and thus social and economic) status of the dead. He uses five classes: I, the upper professional and managerial strata; II, the lesser employers, managers and professions; III, the skilled and blackcoated workers; IV, semi-skilled, including agricultural workers; and V, unskilled labourers. Unfortunately for our purpose here, social class ratios are presented only for age groups of 20 and above. Those for rheumatic fever seem to offer some support for the artisan theory. In age group 20 to 35 the ratios are: 108 for classes I and II, 100 for class III, 106 for class IV, and 84 for class V.

These will not be further discussed, because rheumatic fever is important only in childhood. Several types of heart disease are graded, and chronic endocarditis and valvular disease correspond most closely to the rheumatic group. A steep rise in mortality appears with decline in social status; at 20 to 35 years, the deaths in class V are some 400% of class I.

In middle age, the social gradient flattens, till between 55 and 65, when other than rheumatic causes are increasingly common, the class V mortality is not greatly in excess of that for class I. Occupational risks in themselves are not important; the ratios for married women are almost the same as those for men. It may be noted that the excess of classes IV and V over class III has not altered much but their excess over class I has actually risen since 1910-12. There is no evidence here in favour of the artisan's disease theory; in so far as deaths from rheumatic heart disease can be considered an index of juvenile rheumatism, the findings are very different.

* * * * *

The death rates already cited are averages of England and Wales and include urban and rural, industrial and agricultural experience. The averages are thus made up from widely differing areas, ranging from South-West England to the North East and from Greater London to North and Central Wales. Clearly it is necessary to examine the incidence of juvenile rheumatism in such different settings. The study of these – the social geography of England and Wales – was much simplified when, in 1931, the Registrar-General divided the country into 12 major social and economic regions which bear much more relation to the realities of the social structure of the country than older administrative divisions into counties, boroughs and districts, with their artificial aggregation into North, Midland, South and Wales groups. During the 1930s, for example, the South East, Greater London, the South West and the East were relatively prosperous with a low average of unemployment. South Wales (coalmining), the North East (heavy industry) and Lancashire (cotton) were all abnormally depressed with excessive unemployment rates. Between these economic extremes were the industrial Midland counties and the largely agricultural regions of North Wales, Westmorland and the North and East Ridings of Yorkshire. Such environmental factors can now be observed operating on a large scale and significant local differences need no longer be lost in national averages.

Analysis of mortality from heart disease for ages 5 to 25, the most rheumatic (in our sense) decades, shows that the rates for South-East England, the South West and the Eastern counties are low, for London and the Midlands about average, for the industrial North rather high, and for South Wales throughout in excess of all other regions. In 1930, the Registrar-General stopped listing rheumatic fever in his short tables. Mortality cannot therefore be analysed by the new regions.

The natural climatic factors in themselves seem to be unimportant; as the Registrar-General has pointed out, the climate in South-East and South-West England and in South Wales is very similar. Low-lying and wet East England had the best rate of all. Stevenson (Registrar-General, 1919) noted this in the decennial supplement for 1901-10. Discussing mortality from 'rheumatic fever and rheumatism of the heart', he wrote that the "Fen Counties … return low rates, but the idea of any special association with damp appears to be given up". The mills of God grind slowly.

In 1901-10, mortality at all ages for 'rheumatic fever and rheumatism of the heart', showed similar trends with high rates in the north of England and in Wales.

The figures for rheumatic fever in children (1911-20) likewise closely resemble those found in later years. In 1936-39, there was an all-round improvement, but the glaring regional disparities remained (see also Young, 1921, 1925).

* * * * *

Since Newsholme (1895) emphasised the influence of urbanisation in juvenile rheumatism, this factor has been more or less taken for granted, and relatively little attention has been paid to it. Various investigators have found the incidence greater in the town than in the country. The trend is quite clear and the gradation is steady: mortality rises with increasing density of population.

Study of the mortality rates for rheumatic fever in boys and girls in the regions used by the Registrar-General before 1931 reveals that there is a trend in the expected direction. According to similar analysis for heart disease in children, boys and girls combined, in the Registrar-General's social regions, most of the individual regions show the same unmistakable rise in mortality with increasing urbanisation as was found in all England and Wales; in the North East and the West Riding, the rural rate was about the same as the urban; in Wales, it was worse. It is true that the North East contains some large mining communities, anachronistically labelled 'rural', but in a discussion of density per acre there is no comparing these with the highly urbanised county boroughs, such as Newcastle, Sunderland, Leeds, Sheffield or Bradford.

When the factor of urbanisation is kept constant and areas of similar density are compared, definite discrepancies are discovered. The wide range between the best and worst in all three categories suggests that density of population is not the key factor, and that powerful influences other than urbanisation are operating. At each level, the highest rates are found in South Wales and North England. But the most interesting feature of this regional layout is that mortality from rheumatic fever was greater in the Welsh rural districts than in the urban areas of the whole country or of the North or South; and, in the same way, mortality from (rheumatic) heart disease was higher in the villages of South Wales than in all the big towns, grouped nationally or regionally. We can therefore conclude that, while urbanisation is an unfavourable influence, it is not nearly so decisive as is commonly supposed.

Climate, again, cannot account for the differences found among the northern and southern villages. Rather it seems that the social circumstances in the rural districts of the depressed areas have easily outweighed any advantages, derived from their rural structure, and produced death rates in the North higher than in the big towns of the more prosperous areas, and in South Wales higher than in the worst of the big towns. Danischewsky (quoted by Glover, 1930), discussing the high incidence of acute rheumatism in Moscow, noted that it was still greater in the agricultural villages around the town.

Juvenile rheumatism is not the sole instance where the role of urbanisation has been overrated. In infantile mortality and tuberculosis of young people, for example, the same distribution holds, and the rural districts of the North and Wales register higher mortalities than the much more densely populated cities of other parts of the country.

* * * * *

The death rates for (rheumatic) heart disease in the county boroughs, then, vary widely. To determine what part social factors play in this is not easy. In the first place, there is no ready-made index which assesses the social status of these towns. The levels of unemployment or Poor Law relief are too sensitive to swings of the economic pendulum; Stock's Social Index (Registrar-General, 1936) is not sensitive enough. This index is based on the local distribution of the five social classes. The proportion in classes IV and V (the male semi-skilled and unskilled workers over 14 years) is taken as a measure of local poverty at the time the returns were made, in 1931. Unfortunately, the allocation to the different classes was based on the normal occupation of the individual when in work. No account was taken of unemployment, and consequently the fact that a great number of men and their families had been subjected to a reduction in their standard of living for anything from a few months to many years was not reflected in the social index. However, this index is easily the best available.

Analysis of the death rates for (rheumatic) heart disease in county borough groups for the five years 1929-33 shows a clear trend: the rate for the poorest group of towns is considerably worse than for the most prosperous.

The microclimate (Danischewsky's expression) has also been studied. Housing is usually implicated in the production of juvenile rheumatism by two factors: damp (Miller, 1926) and crowding (Perry and Roberts, 1937; Bach et al, 1939). The degree of overcrowding can be measured both regionally and for the county boroughs from the Ministry of Health Overcrowding Survey. The North East is worst housed by far, being more than twice as crowded as Greater London and four times worse than South Wales. Correlation with mortality from juvenile rheumatism is thus not at all close, and is much clearer for infant mortality and the general death rate in young people.

There is general agreement on the broad issue that juvenile rheumatism is intimately related to an unsatisfactory social environment. Discussion mostly centres on the view that incidence is not determined by the degree of poverty but is highest in the artisan class, and the existence of some particular poverty factor which is primarily responsible for the disease. The approach to these ancient controversies has hitherto been mostly clinical; we have tried the complementary method of statistical analysis which seemed to us more likely to clarify such social medical problems.

We have dealt only with mortality statistics for the very good reason that so few others are available; our ignorance of the morbidity of juvenile rheumatism as of many other major disorders is a long-standing complaint which will not be remedied until periodic health examinations of the whole population are instituted. Schlesinger (1938) has rightly warned against over-emphasis of the fatal issue in this disease; patients do recover from it, or may lead useful lives in spite of it. Mortality does, nevertheless, measure the significance of the condition for the public health, and it sums up the long preceding years of suffering and incapacity. The power of the social factor over mortality from juvenile rheumatism seems established, but it may be objected that the findings cannot simply be applied to the related problems of the incidence of the disease. This difficulty cannot be fully overcome, but analysis of the material meanwhile suggests that the social factor operates principally by enhancing the infection or lowering resistance to it. The other phase of the disease – the cardiac – does not appear to be so strongly affected; neither pregnancy nor occupation, for example, seem to have much influence on the trends which are almost identical for both sexes, for children and young adults. Infection dominates the natural history of this disease – the original tonsillitis, the chronic, relapsing, increasingly severe rheumatism itself, the adventitious respiratory catarrhs. Throughout, the role of the unsatisfactory environment is evident. Coborn (1931) noted that hæmolytic streptococcal throat infections were more common in the unhygienic living conditions of the poor. Hedley (1940) suggests that the more severe forms of rheumatic infection are relatively more common among the very poor. Miller (1934a) observed that no rheumatic child living in his own environment is ever free from the danger of relapse; the relationship of respiratory infections with overcrowding need not be discussed. The thread of infection that runs through the history suggests that the observations made here on mortality may apply with equal emphasis to the earlier stages of the disease as well.

Various field studies – for example, that of the Bristol and Three Counties by Savage (1931) and the MRC investigation in Glasgow and London in 1927 – have analysed poverty in an attempt to discover if any particular constituent was responsible (see also Schlesinger, 1937). The findings have largely been negative. Damp has most persistently been blamed; yet when other conditions are satisfactory, whether in public schools or other institutions, there may be little or no rheumatism. Dutch experience points in the same direction. The specific adverse influence of urbanisation is not proven. A low standard of living, wherever it occurs, whether in town or village, increases the death rate from rheumatic fever and rheumatic heart disease. But poverty is neither the result nor even the necessary associate of greater population density, and to say urbanisation when we mean poverty is no help to clear thinking. Nor do the effects of industrialisation afford an easy explanation. That the fathers of these rheumatic children in the Welsh and northern villages may have been employed at one time or another in the mines cannot directly affect the issue; and the smoke-laden atmosphere of our cities does not apply here. As to overcrowding, our findings have been even less conclusive. The concept of a 'rheumatic stratum' (Miller, 1926), excluding the well-to-do on the one hand and the very poor on the other, received no confirmation. Both regionally and in the big towns, mortality was seen to rise with the degree of poverty.

Climate in this country has little influence. The mortality rates for South-West England and South Wales have already been compared. The contrasts between the rural districts of the north are equally definite. It is interesting that increasing doubt is being cast on the supposed immunity of tropical populations. Swift (1940) discusses the recent and very equivocal literature on this subject. He adds the comment that "crowding, poor housing and poor nutrition seem to play almost as important unfavourable roles in hot as in cold climates".

The upshot seems to be that all these factors – damp and crowding, malnutrition and fatigue, lack of sunshine and holidays, inferior medical care, inadequate clothing and leaky boots – are responsible; that is, the whole life of the underprivileged child. The destruction of the poor is their poverty. In social medicine, such multiple non-specific causation is not unexpected. The first stage in this long history may well be a child constitutionally predisposed to rheumatism. On the whole question of inheritance, there is little substantial evidence. In any case, the disease is seen to be so sensitive to social inequality that emphasis on hereditary influences is premature.

It is still true as in 1927, when Newman wrote, that "no field of preventive medicine offers larger scope for scientific and social investigation than acute rheumatism".

＊ ＊ ＊ ＊ ＊

The morbidity and mortality of juvenile rheumatism have been examined with special reference to the social background of the disease.

Among infections, juvenile rheumatism is probably the greatest cause of sickness and disablement. It causes 2% of all deaths in England and Wales, 10% of all between five and 45. Mortality is declining, although more rapidly in children than young adults. Regionally, and in the county boroughs, the death rate varies widely and rises with the degree of poverty.

Mortality on the whole increases with the density of population; this seems to be a function of the greater poverty in the towns. The depressed rural districts return rates as high as the worst of the big towns.

No evidence was found to suggest that the artisan stratum is particularly prone to the disease. Climate seems of little importance. Correlation with overcrowding was inconclusive.

The facts elucidated strengthen the view that the whole complex of poverty is involved in the production of juvenile rheumatism.

Note
[1] Now rare, phthisis is defined as 'a progressive wasting disease; specifically pulmonary tuberculosis' (*Oxford English Dictionary*).

Health and social change: the example of rheumatic heart disease

The constantly changing interaction of health with society is the base upon which social medicine rests. Many observations have been made to show the influence of social circumstances on birth, life and death. A long and notable series of official reports has related occupational status with mortality rates. These papers, and the studies which have been made upon them by epidemiologists and statisticians, have played no small part in the emergence of what we now call 'social medicine' – or medicine in the matrix of society.

The National Health Survey in the US has yielded comprehensive data on the role of economic factors among the living. In this way, the socially differential mortalities of certain infections, cancers and internal diseases have been determined, and, similarly, the relationship of income levels to certain sickness rates has been identified. In general, it may now be said that the dependence of good health on favourable social circumstances has been amply demonstrated. The reverse is seen to be equally true as our knowledge of the true meaning of a favourable environment continues to expand. This process of interpreting levels of living with states of health has, however, been mainly built up from observations on the nature of 'static' relationships. The human environment, or a somewhat artificial isolate of it, has been correlated with some 'coincident' aspect of health. The basic approach has been, in most cases, one of estimating correspondence or the lack of it between two or more 'static' variants. Often these methods ignore the continuous interplay of social forces and social 'change' with states of wellbeing. Allied to this problem of observing the impact of multiple social change on inconstant states of health is the no less important question of evaluating the relative effects of different environmental factors. Thus we are confronted with a major inquiry: the problem of measuring the response of health to social change. There is no question that, in studying a specific disease, the more searching test of the principles of social medicine is not the observance of a 'static' relationship but a dynamic one – the proof that health *changes* as social conditions *change*. A crude expression of this principle is the wartime behaviour of tuberculosis, cerebro-spinal fever, venereal disease, the dirt diseases, diabetes, anæmia and the action of social stresses on the incidence of gastric and duodenal perforations.

The reduction of such observations to scientific terms has, however, been little attempted.

* * * * *

The first period to be studied selected itself. The boom after the First World War was soon spent and there followed uneasy years in which 'prosperity' obstinately refused to reappear. There is no doubt, however, of the social upheaval caused by the Depression which began late in 1929 and reached bottom about 1932, nor of the slow recovery which then set in. This was an event without parallel in modern history, yet its investigation has been singularly neglected by social medicine. The hypothesis that the health of the community might reflect in its course these changing economic values seems reasonable and worthy of study.

Many indices of economic trends in the years between the wars are available. Taking 1928 as a baseline (100), the value of industrial shares, for example, tumbled by 1932 to 59; the net value of exports to 50. We require, however, a more immediately human measure of the impact of these terrible events on conditions and standards of living. For this purpose, the level of unemployment as it rises and falls is probably a sensitive measure of changing social and economic circumstances. Many social surveys of the 1930s describe in detail the plight of the workless, hovering, it may be for years, on the margin of subsistence. Unemployment meant acute and chronic strain, and the denial of many physical and psychological needs. At no time did unemployment insurance or assistance reach the Beveridge minimum [that is, a subsistence level standard of living]. In the decade 1920-29, an average 10.7% of the insured population were out of work. By 1932, the proportion abruptly doubled to 22.1%. The level of 1920-29 was not regained until 1937. In this paper we have, therefore, used the percentage of unemployment as a measure of changing economic conditions. Nevertheless, we, like other workers in this field, realise its many imperfections. To name only two: the level of rates of benefit and allowances is obviously of importance, so too are changes in the conditions for the receipt of such benefit and allowances. A rise in money payments to the unemployed (this was, in fact, taking place towards the end of the 1930s) and an extension in the classes of persons eligible for assistance are bound to affect the value of the index. Moreover, unemployment only applied to part of the population; we do not know the mortality rates among this section, nor can we measure the influence of the changing level of real wages among the employed population. In short, although it is the best available index for our purpose, it is wise to remember that the incidence of unemployment is still only a very rough and clumsy instrument.

In a previous paper (Morris and Titmuss, 1942), we reviewed the concept of juvenile rheumatism as a 'social' disease, and we demonstrated that its mortality, whether measured by rheumatic fever or heart disease in young people, was affected by the social environment. The association between poverty and a high death rate was clear. There is general agreement, however, on the social origins of the disorder and we have, therefore, chosen it as the first health index to be followed against the changing social background of quasi-normality, decline and recovery. Movements of unemployment levels and associated responses of rheumatic heart disease mortality may reasonably be coupled as cause and effect.

* * * * *

The 12 years under review have been divided into four triennial periods: 1927-29 represents the 'standard' or baseline; 1930-32 the Depression; 1933-35 the beginning of recovery; and 1936-38 the return to what we hesitate to describe as 'normal'. The 83 county boroughs of England and Wales were selected for study mainly because the necessary data were available for these communities. The experience of the 83 individual towns during the 12 years was examined and the mean rates of unemployment and mortality were calculated for each of the four periods. The county boroughs were then arranged in 10 groups lettered A to J. Two considerations decided the grading: the initial 1927-29 level of unemployment (that is, the percentage of insured workers registered as out of work by the Ministry of Labour) and subsequent experience of unemployment from 1930 to 1938.

'Juvenile rheumatism' has been measured by the number of deaths from heart disease in young people aged 5 to 25, both sexes combined, as published annually by the Registrar-General. These terms and 'rheumatic heart disease' will be used interchangeably.

Except in censal years, the detailed figures of the population by ages are not available for individual county boroughs. It was therefore necessary to estimate the numbers at 5 to 25 years in each county borough for the mid-years of three of the triennial periods (that is, for 1928, 1934 and 1937). The data for 1931 were available from the census returns. To ascertain the required figures, the following technique was employed: for each borough, the proportion of the total population in the age range 5 to 25 was computed from the census report for mid-1931. The same proportion was then extracted for the combined county borough population. The Registrar-General supplies the data to allow for similar proportions being calculated for the combined index at mid-1928, 1934 and 1937. The percentage changes for this combined index (1931 = 100) were then computed for the other three mid-years. The results so obtained were then applied to the proportion shown by each borough at 1931. From the revised proportions for each borough, the populations at 5 to 25 for 1928, 1934 and 1937 were calculated by reference to the population at all ages reported by the Registrar-General. It was assumed, therefore, that the rate of change (that is, the upward shift in age structure) in the age composition of each individual borough was the same as that for the combined borough populations. Thus, the differences in age structure among the 83 boroughs shown by the 1931 census were retained for the mid-years 1928, 1934 and 1937. At the same time, this technique took into account the different changes in the total population of each borough (caused by migration, balance of births and deaths, changes in boundaries), as reported by the Registrar-General. Allowance was therefore made for both (a) the initial differences between the proportion of the population aged 5 to 25 in each borough, and (b) the subsequent and different changes in this proportion.

The possibility exists that internal migration, particularly if the migrants are selectively healthy as regards heart disease, may produce distorting effects on local recorded mortalities in the county boroughs. The material bearing on this problem of migration is extremely tenuous. The volume of migration during the period 1927-38 by age, sex, occupation or marital status, so far as it affects the county boroughs, is not known. Nor has the assumption been proved that migration from or to county boroughs is selective. It is, moreover, arguable that an entirely new set of conditions may have obtained during the years of heavy unemployment. The fit may have been better able to obtain local work, and to keep it, in the depressed boroughs while the less fit may have gone in search of work elsewhere (Shannon and Grebenik, 1943). A hint that this may have occurred is provided by F. Grundy (1944), medical officer of health for Luton. During the 1920s and the 1930s, Luton received a great many migrants from depressed areas and experienced, according to Grundy, an abnormally high death rate from tuberculosis among young men.

For a more detailed examination of the whole subject, reference should be made to Hart and Wright (1939) and Lewis-Faning (1938).

During the 12 years under review, 61 county boroughs underwent boundary changes. Of this number, 41 boroughs had one change (regarding changes in a single year as one change), 19 boroughs had two changes and one borough had three changes. The question arose, therefore, whether boundary changes would be likely to influence the death rates. An analysis was therefore made of the boundary and population changes occurring among the 61 boroughs. Out of a total of 10,028 heart disease deaths at ages 5 to 25 in all the county boroughs during 1927-38, only about 20 could have arisen as a result of these factors.

It is clear that the death rates during the 12 years cannot have been affected by any county borough boundary changes.

Table 1: The trend of unemployment and rheumatic heart disease mortality, 1921-38[a]

	1921-23	1924-26	1927-29	1930-32	1933-35	1936-38
England and Wales (all areas)						
Unemployment	14.1	10.4	10.4	20.0	17.4	10.0
Mortality	18.4	16.5	16.6	16.3	16.4	14.2
83 county boroughs						
Unemployment	_[b]	_[b]	11.4	22.3	18.4	13.2
Mortality	20.7	18.8	18.9	19.0	19.2	17.8

[a] The term 'rheumatic heart disease mortality' means the number of deaths (male and female) aged 5 to 25 per 100,000 population aged 5 to 25. The 'unemployment rate' represents the percentage of insured workers (male and female) unemployed (Ministry of Labour's Local Unemployment Index). For groups of years, the average percentage has been computed.

[b] Data not available.

Table 1 depicts the trend of mortality and unemployment in all the county boroughs combined and in England and Wales during 1921–38.

The gap between the mortality of the country as a whole and of the economically more depressed boroughs widened during the difficult years between the wars by 50% and the course of mortality in both was unsatisfactory (after the post-influenzal drop) until 1936–38.

Table 2 sets out the data for unemployment and mortality in our 10 groups of county boroughs.

One of the unhappiest features of the Depression was that towns that could least stand the strain were subjected to the greatest pressure, and this was accompanied by a concentration of unemployment among the poorest paid occupations.

What were the causes which led to the oscillation of the death rates as depicted in Tables 1 and 2? Did changing economic circumstances reflect themselves in a changing mortality from the disorder? Were the oscillations of mortality in sympathy with those

Table 2: Unemployment (U) and rheumatic heart disease mortality (RHD) in the grouped county boroughs, 1927-38[a]

	1927-29		1930-32		1933-35		1936-38	
Gp	U	RHD	U	RHD	U	RHD	U	RHD
A	24.3	20.1	41.6	23.9	41.8	20.7	30.2	24.2
B	13.6	19.3	34.0	19.0	29.5	22.5	21.1	22.0
C	13.7	20.0	31.3	21.1	22.1	23.0	14.8	21.0
D	14.5	21.9	25.9	22.1	24.3	23.2	18.6	20.9
E	11.1	21.1	22.1	19.1	15.0	22.1	11.5	18.6
F	9.7	17.1	18.1	17.9	16.8	18.9	12.0	17.1
G	10.2	17.5	17.7	19.1	14.3	16.8	9.6	15.1
H	11.0	18.1	16.8	16.4	16.0	15.3	11.8	12.7
I	6.3	16.7	14.5	17.2	8.9	16.0	6.2	15.7
J	4.3	11.9	8.8	10.7	8.9	9.2	8.1	9.9

[a] The term 'rheumatic heart disease mortality' means the number of deaths (male and female) aged 5 to 25 per 100,000 population aged 5 to 25. The 'unemployment rate' represents the percentage of insured workers (male and female) unemployed (Ministry of Labour's Local Unemployment Index). For groups of years, the average percentage has been computed.

for unemployment? Viewed as a whole, the one feature of note is the erratic behaviour of the death rates in 1930-32, the years of greatest distress. By 1933-35, a pattern seems to be merging. A to F, the six groups most severely hit by the depression, have by now a higher mortality; and in A to C, the three groups with acute unemployment, this higher mortality persisted to 1936-38. G to J, with death rates already low and additional unemployment of 8.2% or less in 1930-32, all registered a lower death rate in 1933-38. Economic recovery began during 1933-35, a general improvement in mortality in 1936-38. The possibility at once suggests itself that a latent period may be involved in any response of rheumatic heart disease to economic change; in other words, that some time elapses before social changes are reflected in biological effects.

In summing up the picture of these 12 troubled years, the county borough groups have, by 1936-38, taken up a mortality position that conforms less with their original level of unemployment in 1927-29 or with their final level in 1936-38 than with their experience of economic depression and recovery during the whole 12 years. It appears that, relative to each other, the economic vicissitudes they have suffered may have determined their final death rates.

* * * * *

Our present concern is with the reflection of social change in the health of the community. The next step then was to measure the relationship between the amount of change in unemployment and the amount of change in mortality.

A close reading of Table 2 has already suggested that there was a latent period before the full effects of the Depression on mortality rates were observed. We have, therefore, calculated coefficients between the *changes* in unemployment from 1927-29 to 1930-32 and the *changes* in mortality from 1927-29 to 1933-35 to test this suggestion. Similarly, we have correlated the economic change between 1930-32 and 1933-35 with the biological change between 1930-32 and 1936-38.

Table 3 reveals a high positive association between the two movements. Both values are significant. This suggests that, in the evaluation of the effects of economic change on certain types of mortality, the use of a time-lag is warranted.

Table 3: Change correlations – unemployment and 'lagged' mortality

Correlation between change in unemployment	Change in mortality	Grouped data (r)	Ungrouped data (r)
From 1927-29 to 1930-32 with	From 1927-29 to 1933-35	+0.823	+0.333
From 1930-32 to 1933-35	From 1930-32 to 1936-38	0	–0.130

The social indices that are employed today are unsatisfactory in many ways. It may be true that the poverty complex operates as a whole Nevertheless, from knowledge of the manner in which the multiple factors in disease operate with different degrees of intensity in different environments, this would seem to be only partially true. We have considered in this paper three elements: (i) unemployment; (ii) social status, that is, the proportion of the male population aged 14 and over in social classes IV and V at the time of the 1931 census, called the 'Stocks Index of Poverty'; and (iii) the density of room occupation in 1931, called the 'Index of Overcrowding'. (See Registrar-General's 1931 Census Housing Report. The Index of Overcrowding is based on the percentage of the population of each borough living more than two persons per room.) It must suffice to say that, if unemployment is too labile a measure, the other indices are certainly too stable, and in the absence of any data allowing the necessary adjustments to be made, we have assumed that the 1931 indices remained constant throughout the period of this investigation. In other words, the relative differences between the 83 boroughs did not change fundamentally during 1927–38.

The correlation between overcrowding and poverty in the 83 county boroughs during 1931 was +0.459. Similarly, the following variables were associated:

Unemployment and poverty (ungrouped data)	+0.570
Unemployment and overcrowding	+0.442
Mortality and unemployment	+0.563
Mortality and poverty	+0.555
Mortality and overcrowding	+0.340

These correlations confirm what is generally known that the Depression was most heavily concentrated in the worst housed boroughs and in those areas with a high proportion of classes IV and V in their populations.

The next state in this investigation was to submit to further examination the correlations already established between unemployment and mortality by correcting for the influence of the two 1931 social indices – poverty and overcrowding.

Table 4 shows that, as unemployment increased, mortality rose contemporaneously, even when the differences in poverty and overcrowding in the 83 boroughs were neutralised. The relationship is, however, below the required level of significance. But when a mortality lag of three years was introduced – as in the lower half of the table – the values were higher and significant. We tested a six-year lag but found considerably lower values. It seems that the peak relationship is centred between two to four years. This conclusion appears to us to be of some importance from the viewpoint of

Table 4: The relationship between unemployment and mortality and the influence of poverty and overcrowding[a]

Correlation between:	
Change in mortality 1927-29 to 1930-32	
and change in unemployment 1927-29 to	r
1930-32	+0.193
at constant level of poverty index	+0.230
at constant level of overcrowding index	+0.179
at constant level of both indices	+0.216
Change in mortality 1927-29 to 1933-35	
and change in unemployment 1927-29 to	
1930-32	+0.333
at constant level of poverty index	+0.305
at constant level of overcrowding index	+0.319
at constant level of both indices	+0.303

[a] Ungrouped data for the county boroughs, weighted.

examining the interplay of mortality and social change. It is not, of course, a revolutionary suggestion – that mortality changes should lag behind depression or prosperity – but it must be said that hitherto such techniques have not been widely exploited.

We have, up to this point, established a relationship between unemployment and mortality changes during the depression phase of the 12 years. What is, so far, less clear is the effect of declining unemployment on mortality during the recovery phase. This may be due to the impossibility of carrying the investigation beyond 1938. On the other hand, the suggestion that overcrowding and poverty may have slowed down mortality improvement is worth examining further. In Table 5, we have computed the correlations between mortality changes and the 1931 levels of the poverty and overcrowding indices.

In the first periods examined, when the overall death rate in the county boroughs was rising, there is no significant association between mortality change and the indices in question. On the other hand, we found that there was a positive and significant correlation between unemployment change (1927-29 to 1930-32) and both social indices. We also found that there was a positive – and again significant –

Table 5: Mortality change and the social indices in the county boroughs during 1927-38 (ungrouped data)

Correlation between: Change in mortality	Index of poverty (r)	Overcrowding held constant (r)	Index of overcrowding (r)	Poverty held constant (r)
1927-29 to 1930-32	−0.037	+0.080	+0.074	+0.102
1927-29 to 1933-35	+0.139	+0.104	+0.101	+0.043
1930-32 to 1933-35	+0.181	+0.188	+0.032	−0.058
1930-32 to 1936-38	+0.784	+0.728	+0.690	+0.599

correlation between unemployment change and lagged mortality. Thus, with the existing incidence of poverty and overcrowding held constant, it appears that rising unemployment was, at least partly, responsible for the latent rise in mortality.

We now turn to the second phase: the period of declining unemployment. Here there was a close association between the rise and fall in unemployment and a significant relationship between unemployment fall, and both poverty and overcrowding. In other words, those boroughs with excessive overcrowding and a high proportion of unskilled and semi-skilled workers upon whom fell the heaviest burden of unemployment benefited most from the later decline in depression. But did this fall in unemployment result in a fall in mortality? The answer is no; we found no significant correlation. The highly significant and positive correlations between mortality change 1930–32 to 1936–38 and both social indices indicate that these factors of social status and overcrowding retarded the improvement that might have been expected with the lightening of unemployment. In other words, heavy unemployment superimposed on overcrowding and low economic status produced higher mortality; when unemployment lifted somewhat, these factors of bad housing and low social status assumed *greater* relative importance and prevented the expected decline in mortality. Their relative influence was much more static during the 12 years (1927–38). Neither the county borough distribution of social status nor of housing densities fluctuated as violently over this period as did the factor of unemployment.

* * * * *

Our observations invite the comment that they make a disconcerting postscript to many assurances on the unimportance of the Depression to the people's health. Similarly, they may be worth examining as a measure of the insulation afforded by pre-war social services. In general, it can be said that the evidence now gathered re-emphasises the principle that 'the public health is purchasable'. In particular, the conclusion of this investigation strengthens the concept that juvenile rheumatism is a social disease, an 'ill bred by poverty'.

Our immediate concern is with the manner in which economic changes are reflected in sensitive vital statistics. The period 1927–38 was a time of violent social flux. In the Depression of 1930–32, the death rate from rheumatic heart disease responded in sympathy with economic trends. That the trend of mortality was a response to undercurrents in conditions of living (as expressed through the level of unemployment) and that the rise in unemployment produced at least part of the rise in mortality, is a logical conclusion from our knowledge of the power which social influences wield in the genesis of juvenile rheumatism. During the phase of recovery, the association of the course of mortality and the movement of unemployment was no longer significantly discernible. Unemployment fell rapidly in just those towns where previously it had risen sharply; the changes in mortality were, however, in slower motion and, in any case, cannot be pursued beyond 1938. The weakness of the association during such of the recovery period as could be brought under review was thus not unexpected. Not only did the problem of the time-lag in the recovery phase intervene but it became clear that, as the importance of unemployment declined, the twin evils of economic status and bad housing were seen to be buttressing the death rate. As the waves of unemployment subsided, they revealed the peaks of other adverse factors in the social environment. These retrogressive factors, still as effective as hitherto, had, however, been temporarily overshadowed by the catastrophes of 20-50% unemployment.

So far as juvenile rheumatism is concerned, amidst all the 'multiple factors' that produce this disorder, the biological must not be forgotten. Clinical experience of juvenile rheumatism suggests a progressive decline in its severity; it is an 'obsolescent disease' (Glover, 1930). Such diminishing virulence (or increasing immunity) are not infrequent variations in the natural history of infectious processes. From 1924 to 1935, however, this decline in juvenile rheumatism was not manifest in the course of the death rate from heart disease. There is little material on morbidity to compare with the valuable mortality data provided by the Registrar-General, although Bach et al (1939) reported a fall of almost two thirds in the *incidence* of heart disease among London school children during these 12 years. It would seem more than a very remarkable coincidence that only with a *turn* in social conditions for the better – even if this 'better' was only pre-slum 'normality' – did this clinical fact become true once again of the death rate as well. And over about one third of the population (the total county borough group), which registered a rate of Depression conspicuously higher than that for the national average, the almost stationary mortality record of England and Wales during 1924-35 was translated into a slight but clearly perceptible increase in the death rate. When this was broken down, we saw that it contained widely varying reactions in harmony with the changing levels of unemployment in the individual and grouped county boroughs. The increase in mortality was much more definite in those towns with a considerable increase in unemployment; in the others there was, in fact, an equally definite fall. With the lightening in unemployment, there was a belated decline in mortality in 1936-38, greater in the country as a whole than in the harder pressed county boroughs.

Migration was not, we consider, an important factor in producing these mortality trends. Not only did the death rates (per 100,000 population aged 5 to 25) rise, but the number of deaths increased. For instance, in the heavily depressed county borough of Gateshead, the number of deaths for the four triennial periods were 26, 32, 33 and 36. Selective migration could hardly have produced this result.

The irregular response in 1930-32 provokes curiosity. There was an indecisive period before a design came clearly into focus. That such a lag occurred, even with a convulsion so violent as the one we have been studying, is very suggestive. The key to it may lie in two directions. Unemployment in the 1930s meant malnutrition and squalor, not starvation and exposure; juvenile rheumatism is a malady whose natural history runs a long and tangled course. On both accounts, it is not surprising that its death rate was not as closely superimposed on the course of unemployment as the historic waves of pestilence on famine. The economic forces were no longer so free and the results – in terms of juvenile rheumatism – gathered momentum more slowly and were of smaller intensity, although in the end they stood out as clearly.

The interaction of the 'temporary' social factor of mass unemployment with two of the more permanent features of pre-war Britain – the number of poorly paid workers and the degree of overcrowding – is noteworthy. During the Depression, the onrush of unemployment was the dominant environmental element. As the tide of unemployment receded, the inexorable social facts of 'regular' poverty and crowded homes easily reasserted themselves and established control again over mortality from disorders like juvenile rheumatism. With the outbreak of war, and full and higher paid employment achieved, the stage was set for a further improvement in this social health index. The findings of Glover (1943) are highly apposite. The remarkable decline in mortality since 1939 is in complete accord with the findings of this investigation. We fully realise that there are other agencies which contribute to the onset and course of the disease. But some of these – the genetic factor, for instance – cannot be measured in an investigation of this kind. It must not be overlooked, moreover, that we have not been studying morbidity indices in this paper; we have been concerned with the killing agencies. It is as well that, at the conclusion of an investigation of this type, such things should be borne in mind. Statistical relationships expressed in the employment of correlation coefficients have their limitations. Such limitations should be remembered even if every sentence that is written does not contain a qualifying participle.

* * * * *

In the county boroughs of England and Wales, changing socioeconomic circumstances during the Depression of 1930-32 (as measured by the level of unemployment) were reflected *subsequently* in the level of mortality from rheumatic heart disease at ages 5 to 25.

'Mass' unemployment, while it lasted, appeared as the dominant social influence, and temporarily assumed control of the course of the mortality studied.

With the partial lifting of the Depression, the more permanent adverse factors – such as bad housing and the proportion of low paid workers – were no longer overshadowed and reassumed their influential role in determining the course of the death rate. These factors retarded the decline in mortality which set in towards the end of the 1930s.

This investigation has established a relationship between changing economic levels and a changing mortality rate. In the disease specifically studied in this paper, it has been further shown that the association is strengthened when a mortality lag of three years is introduced. In terms of its relative influence as a factor in the total social environment, mass unemployment has been demonstrated to be of considerable importance. When unemployment fell to around 15%, the factors of low economic status and overcrowding were seen to be exercising some weight in determining the course of mortality. After the outbreak of war in 1939, the death rate from heart disease between the ages of 5 and 25 fell to a remarkable extent, despite the fact that the housing situation in the country steadily deteriorated. Full employment and higher wages were factors which, judged by the lessons of this study, obviously affected the course of mortality.

A further product of this investigation is the manner in which it extends and deepens the concept of juvenile rheumatism as a social disease and, incidentally, as a most sensitive index of social conditions. By the employment of such methods as explained in this paper, social medicine might eventually frame a series of laws governing the manifold dynamic interactions of health with society.

War and disease

Disease has always reaped a rich harvest in time of war. It has done so quietly and insidiously under cover of the conditions created by war because dirt and insanitary conditions are inseparable from fighting. The louse and carriers of typhus, the enteric fevers and other diseases are determined camp followers. It has been said with truth that the real conquerors of the Roman Empire were not the Goths and the Vandals, but malaria and plague. Disease has, in the past, settled a good many wars, and the victors have not always been the strongest military power. Even when modern artillery arrived, disease still claimed the most victims. In the American Civil War, the Federal Army lost twice as many men from disease as from wounds. In the Crimean War, mortality from dirt diseases among the fighting men was immensely high. The real hero of that war was Florence Nightingale who reduced mortality from wounds and disease among the soldiers by two thirds. Yet we did not take those lessons fully to heart. We still thought in terms of the dramatic – shell fire and the bayonet. In the Boer War [1899-1902], over 14,000 British soldiers died of disease, as against 8,000 who were killed in battle or died of wounds.

But it was not until the last war [the First World War, 1914-18] that we realised how greatly the civilians are also involved in the battle against disease. Insufficient food, overcrowding, poor clothing, long hours of work – all these things reduce resistance to disease among the people at home. Let us see how the civilians, as compared with the soldiers, fared in the last war. Among the British forces, 550,000 were killed or died of wounds and disease. These men are remembered by their country, but how many people know that the war directly caused the deaths of 340,000 civilians from disease? For every 10 fighting men who died, seven civilians were carried off by disease caused by the war. In Europe, it was much worse than that. Germany lost another quarter of a million civilians from tuberculosis alone. In the whole world, disease claimed 10 million people, many more than the total population of Australia and New Zealand [in 1943].

We cannot have a better illustration of the growing interdependence of all nations than the effects of modern war on disease. For one thing, easier and faster transport all over the earth can lead to the rapid spread of epidemics; witness the movement of the influenza outbreak in 1919. This epidemic had its roots in the conditions created by the war in Europe, but the disease did not confine itself to the warring countries in Europe. For instance, more people died of war influenza in India than the total battle losses of all belligerents between 1914 and 1918. Even some of the remote islands of the Pacific suffered more heavily than the people of Britain. One quarter of the population of Samoa died from influenza. They would not have died but for the war, so there can be no neutrals in the war against disease. The louse does not recognise frontiers; tuberculosis ignores race and language. Neutrality in this war [the Second World War, 1939-45], by lengthening the period of fighting, must mean greater mortality from disease among the neutrals.

We knew, from the lessons of history, that when this war came, one of our greatest enemies would be disease; that, at every turn, in the home, in the street and in the hospital, the battle would have to be relentlessly waged. The dangers in 1939 were far greater than in 1914. The bomber had increased the opportunities for disease to spread. It was clear that, if we did not control the situation, the microbe and parasite would control us. The bomber, with high explosive and incendiary bombs, would blast a way for the germ and for the barrack-room disease, such as spotted fever. Well, we were not far wrong; this is what happened. High explosive has burst open the mains and blended water with sewage. Gas mains have been punctured and flames have risen 50 feet. The bombs have shaken up the dust and dirt of centuries in London and other cities and it has got into our clothes, our homes and our food. Worse than that, however, is the fact that people have been driven to crowd together in basements, shelters and tube stations. Hundreds of thousands of people – old and young, healthy and sick, dirty and clean – have been forced at times to spend 15 hours out of every 24 in ill-ventilated holes and tunnels. For nearly a year, a very large section of the people lived in this way. Today [1943] conditions are better, but for four years we have had to sleep in blacked-out, badly ventilated rooms. Many of us have to spend all our working hours in bricked-up offices and factories. In too many parts of the country, the housing shortage is so acute that beds are never cold. Two workers will rent one bedroom and the day shift takes over the bed when the night shift goes to work. The crowding together in buses and trains, theatres and cinemas is just as bad. There is one town as large as Perth, which started the blitz with 35 cinemas. When Goering had done his best, there were only two left.

In most of the large cities, we are living on top of one another. The war has boxed us up. In factory, office and workshop, all available space is in use. Empty flats and houses are almost impossible to obtain. In London and other cities, we have to wait patiently for crowded buses, trains and meals. We eat and travel with, so to speak, a strange elbow in our back. We sleep, on fire-watching nights, to the accompaniment of the noise of a stranger. We shut out the air and we only see the stars when we are on civil defence duty. It isn't pleasant, but it is war. The danger here, where there is so little room to turn round – mentally as well as physically – is the greater chance of disease spreading. The less room that we have in which to live, the greater the opportunity for the microbe. Those are the environmental risks of modern war, and they are greatest in the congested industrial centres.

But housing, air, sun and pure water – these are only one aspect of the battle. There are other sectors of this campaign of which food is the most important. And we now know that it is the composition of the diet which is so vital for health. During the Russo-Japanese War [1904–05], there were two million cases of beri-beri in the Japanese army but none in the navy. The rations were about the same, except that the sailors' diet included 10oz of whole barley, and those 10oz made all the difference. The collapse of the Italians at Caporetto in October 1917 was due in part to the fact that the Italian army ration was 20% lower than that of the British, French and German. There is a saying in the East expressive of food deficiencies, 'It is better to walk than to run; it is better to stand than to walk; it is better to lie than to stand; it is better to sleep than to wake; it is better to die than to live'. It is a way of expressing, in other words, progressive vitamin B1 deficiency. It contributed to the collapse of Germany in 1918 and affected many of the armies. Today, we see that the civilian ration is as good for maintaining health as the army ration.

So far, I have given some examples of how disease can turn the scales of war and I have described how the bomber has opened up vast new territories for the germ and the virus to attack. Yet, after nearly four years of war, Britain's health record is good. How is that? Have we conquered disease or are we only holding it at bay? In a small country like Britain, with a highly elaborate and centralised system of health and sanitary control, the bomber could have wrecked administration in a short time. So the first step that we took was to decentralise our machine for the prevention and cure of disease. This was an important act and out of it has developed a new pattern for the future. Mothers can now leave the cities and have their babies in maternity homes in the country. Thousands of under-fives are living in country hostels; some of them are orphans, while in other cases both parents are working or are in the forces. The sick and wounded are sent to country hospitals to recuperate. Since the beginning of the war, the government has helped three million people to leave London and other bombed areas for a time. On the mental plane, the knowledge that evacuation was always open has proved to be an immensely useful safety valve. And, when we are fighting strain and weariness and all the minor irritations of war, safety valves are good things to have. One of the most surprising facts about this war is the general absence of nervous breakdowns or war neuroses. All the psychiatrists predicted a collapse in mental health. Instead, we have had a decline in the number of cases.

In addition to these wise administrative measures, we have called in science and the techniques of planning to aid us on the home front. Supplementary feeding, vitamin concentrates, fruit juices, the soya bean, fortified bread, communal feeding and a host of other measures have helped to sustain health. Then we have had the new drugs – the sulphonamides – which have already saved thousands of lives. But the story of the advances made by medical science in this war is a long one. The use of dried blood, mass radiography, new methods of cleansing air-raid shelters, improvements in war surgery, new treatment of shell blast, new knowledge of the habits of the itch-mite, are all part of the story. Never in so short a space of time has such a revolution been wrought in the treatment of so many diseases. All this and, perhaps most important of all, full employment and regular wages, have held disease at bay. But it is never far away. For instance, by the end of 1942, 11,000 more people died from tuberculosis in England and Wales over the peacetime figure. They would not have died but for the war. This is a small increase compared with the last war, but it is a warning that we must remain on guard. We must go on thinking in terms of prevention; of building up resistance to weariness – the forerunner of disease – until, after victory, we can all have a long, sunlit holiday.

The National Health Service

Commentary: John R. Ashton

Michael Moore, bête noir of the proponents of the recent war in Iraq, has proposed a rule that countries should not be allowed to wage war on other countries unless they know where they are. He bases this on the finding by the *National Geographic* magazine that 80% of Americans did not know where Iraq is. Yet how many health policy makers of the past 25 years have known and understood the origins and dynamics of health and health services so clearly and beautifully mapped out in such incisive plain English by Richard Titmuss? Surely nobody should be allowed to mess about with, or wage war on, the British National Health Service (NHS) unless they can demonstrate a proper understanding of the range of issues laid bare, clearly and in depth in these writings.

* * * * *

Titmuss's essays and lectures on the NHS remain as pertinent today as when they were written almost 50 years ago. They cover the origins of the NHS in the Wartime Emergency Medical Service; trends and dilemmas in social policy and medical care; a consideration of the confusing and complex structural issues underlying the NHS; and some intriguing perspectives on general practice. Finally, and not least, there are observations on the ethics and economics of medical care.

In his sharp and perceptive analyses, speaking down the decades, Titmuss has something valuable to contribute on most contemporary health policy themes, and the resonances are sometimes uncannily powerful. Beginning with a consideration of the organisation of the Wartime Emergency Medical Service, his discussion of how war has shaped and impacted on health policy and health services is particularly poignant in the aftermath of the destruction of the World Trade Center in New York, the American 'war on terrorism', and the controversial wars in the Middle East. As Titmuss reminds us, the Boer War (1899–1902) revealed the appalling state of industrial working-class youth after a sustained period of unmoderated free market and imperial ambition, a class so degraded and having benefited so little from capitalism that it was unfit to defend the British Empire against its competitors. The result was a range of preventive public health measures, including the provision of free school meals and the establishment of the school health service. From the First World War

(1914-18) came the creation of the Ministry of Health, developments for the care of mothers and young children, and the establishment of clinical services to diagnose and treat sexually transmitted disease. And, from the Second World War (1939-45), the Emergency Medical Service put in place the framework and the structure, with all its contradictions, of the evolution of the National Health Service in 1948. This, apparently a symbol of war socialism, was carried over into the great Attlee reforming government of 1945, and was a manifestation of the huge generosity of spirit and altruism of a generation returning from war – determined to invest in the future to prevent another recession producing the economic conditions in which war would flourish. Ironically, one of the early effects of the attacks on the World Trade Center and concern about bioterrorism has been a renewed commitment to fundamental public health in the guise of health protection (germs, chemicals, disasters and externally derived threats to what the Americans now call 'homeland security'). We had known for over 20 years that our public health services were no longer fit for the purpose. To paraphrase the former Conservative British Cabinet Minister, Michael Heseltine, commenting on what was needed to do something about the decline of the first port of the British Empire, Liverpool, "It took a riot" – or, in this case, the demolition of the World Trade Center – to do something about public health.

The principal components of the Emergency Medical Service were the voluntary and municipal hospitals. This two-tier system of medical care is real food for thought for those who think that foundation hospitals are a panacea. Shortages of surgeons, worn-out administrative boundaries, and arguments about the right size for a hospital abounded. For many patients, transfer from a well-resourced voluntary hospital to a 'pest house', municipal hospital was a sentence of death. Yet all was not well in the voluntary hospitals either and, as Titmuss observes, a bad doctor will still be a bad doctor, however excellent the hospital and its equipment. The peculiar situation of London tantalised then, as it had Chadwick 100 years earlier, and as it does today; we have to ask the question, what benefit has it brought to the people of London to have such a concentration of teaching hospitals and medical research? The 'inverse care law' associated with the work of South Wales GP, Julian Tudor Hart, is clearly evidenced here, with seven times as many family doctors in Kensington as in South Shields. Reading Richard Titmuss on the NHS, I am reminded that having waiting lists is a civilised thing and not a managerial failure; waiting lists are a way of making unmet need explicit so that priorities can be decided. We have no idea what the waiting lists are in the USA, where something in the region of 40 million Americans have no medical care.

Writing at the end of 2003, I am particularly interested in the notion of one standard for a service providing care for 50 million people over and above the founding mothers' and fathers' vision of equal access for equal need, free at the time of use. There has never been one standard and it is clear from Richard Titmuss's work that what we got in 1939 was two hospital services imposed on two hospital systems: one centrally controlled and financed, the other not – out of which came the system based on 14 Regional Hospital Boards. Recent years have seen this tier of public administration juggled with, first down to eight and then nine NHS Regional Offices, then a short-lived four Directorates for Health and Social Care, and at the moment, pending the advent of foundation hospitals, 28 Strategic Health Authorities. While this has been going on, government departments other than the Department of Health have been lining themselves up with the new Government Offices for the Regions, of which there are nine, in anticipation of further devolution of government to the regional level for the first time. We could well be anticipating new-style 'Regional Health Boards' mapped on to the devolved Regional Assemblies at some time in the future.

Titmuss's reflections on trends in social policy take us into wider fields altogether. Here he explores the conditions of general practice and the increasing impact of science. The vexed issue of the paper tiger threat, 'the nanny state', receives due attention. In the person of Dicey (1905), we hear that, for the state to act in the interests of "the best ascertained laws of health" meant, to him, a grave threat to liberty for such action signified, "government for the good of the people by experts, or officials who know or think they know, what is good for the people better than either any non-official person or than the mass of the people themselves". Suffice to say that Titmuss takes these arguments apart with an impressive thoroughness. Politicians who run for cover at the mere mention of 'the nanny state' would do well to listen.

The two Welshmen, David Lloyd-George and Aneurin Bevan, who were not afraid of 'nanny state' allegations, left the British this abiding legacy. From Titmuss's writings, we learn, too, that by 1905 Freud was beginning to exert his influence on health policy and that, with the beginnings of rational therapy, diagnosis was beginning to matter. The profession of medicine was undergoing important changes and an understanding of the nature of the doctor–patient relationship was beginning its long journey to the fore. As Titmuss says (see page 75), "These movements – scientific, professional and economic – were shifting the emphasis in matters of health and disease from the situation to the person; from the environment to the individual; from the public health officer to the general practitioner".

The big question for us is where today's megatrends – increased life expectancy, the conquest of many diseases, information technology and a revolt by the laity against professional hegemony – are leading.

Whither hospitals and who is in the ascendancy? I am prompted to speculate as to whether today's epidemic of obesity may have the same impact on social policy as the Boer War 100 years ago.

Titmuss reminds us of what some may have forgotten: that the original structure of the NHS owed more to the opinion of doctors than to political and public opinion. In many ways, Lloyd-George in 1911 saved the GPs from the Friendly Societies and the insecurity of contract practice. There is scope here for a closer examination of the current infatuation with North American Health Maintenance Organizations. There are well-kept secrets, such as the fact that GPs doubled their salaries in 1911; the middle classes were among the principal beneficiaries of the NHS in 1948, having been excluded in 1911 in part because of their excessive demands on care; and the fact that the NHS has led to the medical profession becoming even more of a self-replicating social elite than it was before. Titmuss's opinion that the accountability of medicine to society has never been adequately addressed is still relevant today.

Taken from his *Essays on 'The welfare state'* (Titmuss, 1963b), the chapters on NHS structure and general practice revisit some of the previous territory. However, as always with Titmuss, the sweep tends to take you by surprise. He makes comparisons between British and American attitudes to health – something which today is even more relevant. "For Americans", argues Titmuss, "good health is seen as a prerequisite for the success of the personality and simultaneously as a necessary condition for the enjoyment and exploitation of success". He comments that each distinctive culture gets the medical priesthood it wants, which explains the co-dependency of Americans on their doctors.

Too many doctors? Not enough doctors? Too expensive? Not well enough funded? In the early 1950s, a distinguished Cambridge economist (Guillebaud Committee, 1956) reviewed

> The present and prospective cost of the National Health Service … to suggest means whether by modifications in organisation or otherwise of ensuring the most effective control and efficient use of such Exchequer funds as may be made available; to advise how, in view of the burdens of the Exchequer arising charge upon it can be avoided while providing for the maintenance of an adequate service; and to make recommendations.

Exactly 50 years later, a distinguished banker (Sir Derek Wanless) does something similar, coming up with a 'fully engaged scenario' to tackle the determinants of health across Whitehall, with an enhanced, cross-boundary focus on prevention and especially on obesity, diabetes and smoking.

Wartime neglect of the fabric of British hospitals meant that the 1950s was catch-up time; today, with Private Finance Initiatives after 20 years of underfunding, the parallels jump out at you. In 1944, 80% of the population provided 5% of the medical students; today, something like 70% of medical students have professional parents. At least one thing seems to have gone: when I was applying to medical school in 1965, each of the London schools had a similar form which enquired, before getting into rugby and cricketing prowess, whether your father was a doctor or a vicar and, if the former, whether he [*sic*] had qualified there. Recruitment to medical school continues to fish in limited pools with selection methods that fall short of modern commercial or other public sector practice.

Turning finally to Titmuss on 'The ethics and economics of medical care' (Part 2, Chapter Five), my feeling is that this is what he may have been most passionate about. "I happen to believe", he says , "that the conflict between professional ethics and economic man should be reduced as far as humanly possible (in the social situation in which the doctor finds himself today)". Titmuss certainly takes issue with a pamphlet, *Health through choice*, by the American D.S. Lees (1961), in which the author argues for the invisible hand of the market to operate for health services as in classical economic theory; the function of consumers is to choose, bargain and buy – not to organise supply. Choice is currently a fashionable notion in health care. Titmuss has plenty to say on the subject. This, like much of his writing on the NHS, should be required reading in the corridors of power.

Towards a national hospital service

The direct and indirect consequences of war have profoundly influenced the development of the nation's medical services. War in general has provided clinical and surgical material for experimentation on a grand scale and has imbued society upon each outbreak with a fresh interest in health.

Because war means the organisation of killing and wounding, it must also mean the organisation of services to repair and heal. The Crimean War [1853-56] led, through the work of Florence Nightingale, to the creation of a nursing profession and to improvements in hospital administration; recruitment for the Boer War [1899-1902] revealed defects which directed attention to the physique and health of children and stimulated the provision of school meals and a school medical service, while the First World War [1914-18] gave birth to the Ministry of Health, spurred on the movement for the care of mothers and young children, and led to a scheme for the diagnosis and treatment of venereal disease. These were not new ideas; the momentum of war spread and quickened a trend towards social altruism and crystallised within the nation demands for social justice.

The accumulated lessons, both good and bad, which emerged from the experience of war to shape in peacetime the structure of medical care, had been generally acquired after war had broken out and in the process of fighting it. But this is by no means true of the Second World War [1939-45]. The frame and pattern of the hospital services at the end of the war were due as much – if not more – to the kind of war that was expected as to the kind of war that happened.

The estimates of the Air Staff, the translation of these into figures of casualties and hospital beds, and the prevailing mood of fear and alarm about the character of a future war had largely determined, by the end of 1938, the way in which the medical services of the country were to be organised eventually. The outline of Britain's first attempt to create a national hospital service was clearly pictured before the war began.

* * * * *

The dominant feature of the pre-war situation was the existence of two distinct and contrasting hospital systems: voluntary and municipal. Both had grown up without a plan. Their origins and histories were dissimilar; they were differently organised and financed and, in some respects, they catered for different sections of the population. Of all the hospitals in England and Wales (excluding mental and convalescent homes and hospitals run by the defence services), less than half the number, and less than one third of the total beds, were under voluntary management; the rest were controlled by local authorities.

The Ministry faced a rigid and conservative social institution. First, there existed a multiplicity of individualistic voluntary hospitals, ranging from the great teaching hospitals to the small, debt-ridden institutions sometimes over-proud of their operating theatres but often short of surgical specialists. Second, there were the local authority hospitals, tied to out-worn boundaries, receivers of all the unwanted and uninteresting 'chronic' cases, still flavoured with the stigma of the Poor Law, and often badly equipped and accommodated in large, prison-like buildings. Somehow or other the Ministry had to bring together these rival systems, and to create, out of "the varying and independently provided hospital facilities" (Ministry of Health, 1944, Cmd 6502, p 56), a national organisation for the care and treatment of all raid casualties.

Within each of these systems, there were remarkable differences. Some were largely charitable, while others were chiefly financed by weekly contributions from certain groups of workers; the miners of South Wales, for example, mainly provided some of the hospitals in that part of the country. The evolution, then, of a thousand and more voluntary hospitals was very diverse; their standards of performance, their staffing and equipment, and their debts and endowments varied immensely in 1939.

Because of their larger size and greater number of beds, the general hospitals and institutions provided by local authorities formed – in terms of accommodation – the backbone of the emergency hospital scheme. A substantial number of these institutions had developed from the early poorhouses, where those without means were made to work under harsh conditions. Originally, these institutions had not been provided for ill people, but, with the passage of time, they became more and more responsible for the old and destitute sick, for chronic, incurable and senile patients. This, their main function in 1939, was left to them by the voluntary hospitals.

There is much evidence concerning the selection of patients by voluntary hospitals, the resulting accumulation of particular types of sickness and groups of people in publicly owned institutions, and the ill-effects of this segregation. A report issued by King Edward's Hospital Fund and the Voluntary Hospitals Committee for London (1945) drew attention to the practice whereby voluntary hospitals exercised "their discretion over the admission of these patients (the chronic sick) and having admitted them transfer them to municipal hospitals". During 1935-37, some 27,000 patients were transferred by voluntary hospitals to general hospitals provided by the London

County Council. This practice meant for many old people – particularly in the provinces where hospitals rarely touched the high standards achieved by London – a sentence of death. The municipal hospital or institution often became known as a receiver of incurables, and those that entered its doors felt that they were being "put away" (Institute of Almoners, 1946).

Almost without exception, accommodation for these chronic sick (including large numbers of people with cancer) was available only in public assistance hospitals and institutions which often did not provide "either the physical or mental amenities to be found in even the most ordinary well conducted domestic dwelling" (Ministry of Health, 1945a, reporting on the 1938 position in Yorkshire). A departmental survey of public assistance institutions in a county within 50 miles of London described them, just before the war, as "pesthouses".

After the passage of the Local Government Act of 1929, empowering the major local authorities to appropriate public assistance institutions and to enter the field of general hospital provision, the differences in standards and performance of work among municipal hospitals widened considerably. This new function was not a statutory duty. In consequence, some authorities forged ahead and provided first-class hospitals with a complete range of specialist departments and staff, while other authorities were content to maintain their institutions as Poor Law infirmaries. In one county near London, described in an official report as feudal and parsimonious, the word of one or two local people was often more powerful than the council itself, while in a south-western county (Ministry of Health, 1945b, reporting on the 1938 position), the nursing staff of public assistance institutions had to start washing the inmates at three to four o'clock in the morning because they were so short-handed. In seven out of 52 institutions admitting sick persons in the south-west region, not one trained nurse was employed. Over the whole of England and Wales, some 70,000 beds in 140 hospitals were being maintained under public health powers just before the war, while nearly 60,000 more in 400 hospitals and institutions were still administered under the Poor Law (Ministry of Health, 1944, Cmd 6502).

The age, structural condition and equipment of a large number of municipal – and voluntary – hospitals was unsatisfactory. Many of the country's hospitals were erected for other purposes and at a time when ideas about the treatment of disease were quite different from those prevailing in the 1930s. One report after another spoke of large old-fashioned wards, out-of-date kitchens, poor and insufficient equipment, inadequate or non-existing laboratories, ugly prison-like buildings, and old and dilapidated structures. Of 21 institutions for the chronic sick existing on the eve of war in South Wales and Monmouthshire (Ministry of Health, 1945c), nine were over 100 years old, eight over 50 years, two more than 40 years old, while the remaining two were put up in 1904 and 1908. All were built as workhouses for paupers. The surveyors classified all hospitals (voluntary and municipal but excluding tuberculosis and mental institutions) and found that, out of a total of 7,945 beds, 3,855 – or nearly one half – were in premises graded as totally unfit to be used as hospitals.

But these considerations of structure, condition and equipment were overshadowed by the crucial problem: the number and quality of the medical and nursing staff. The organisers of the emergency medical service foresaw in 1939 an acute shortage in quantity; there would not be, if the expected number of air raid casualties materialised, enough doctors, specialists, nurses and hospital technicians. There was less recognition then of shortages in relation to the existing needs of the sick population.

Part of the explanation of these pre-war shortages was to be found in the way medical resources were distributed. A few areas of the country and a small section of the people were abundantly served with medical and nursing skill, but in many places, especially the economically depressed areas, there were widespread shortages. This was very true of expert medical skill.

The uneven distribution of medical skill in relation to needs was made worse by another characteristic of the pre-war hospital services: an uneconomic distribution of cases to beds. A complicated case would often receive treatment in a hospital with neither the staff nor the equipment to treat it, while a simple case would occupy a bed in a hospital with a high standard in staff and equipment. According to hospital survey reports, published by the Ministry of Health in 1945-46, the tendency of some consultants to maintain personal waiting lists while others had vacant beds presented a problem of a rather different order. The co-existence of two hospital systems was one of the fundamental causes. Yet another was traceable to an uncoordinated and parochial ambulance service composed of many different types of ambulances equipped with stretchers which were not interchangeable.

All the evidence that had accumulated by 1945 showed that there was a general shortage of hospital beds for sick people before the war. It was on top of this 'normal' shortage that the abnormal wartime shortage – an immense one, according to all forecasts – would be imposed.

Pre-war deficiencies in hospital accommodation – both for general and special needs – were due to a variety of causes. Some of these, such as the maldistribution of consultants and the restrictive practices of voluntary and municipal hospitals, have already been mentioned. Others were to be found in a shortage of nursing staff, defects in the organisation of hospital work, lack of proper equipment and the tendency for beds in large hospitals to be allocated to separate units or firms, working more or less independently (Gardner and Witts, 1946). Above all, many voluntary hospitals were facing financial crises, while local authorities had entered the field of general hospital provision at a time when financial economy was the watchword. Apart, therefore, from a few of the wealthier local authorities, municipal hospitals were, up to the outbreak of war, short of money. That is one reason why, when the time came to organise the emergency scheme, many municipal hospitals and public-assistance institutions were found to contain in their general wards an unholy and unhygienic collection of nursing mothers, infants with gastroenteritis, healthy new-born babies, and aged and chronically sick women.

These then were the kind of problems which the government faced when the planning of a wartime hospital service began. This was the basic stuff, which could not be swept away overnight and replaced with brand new hospitals, new equipment and new staff.

*****

In 1939, the question of organising hospital provision for war victims was approached as a separate and self-contained issue. It was agreed that the existing pattern of hospital organisation should be preserved for the civilian population, but for those patients, regarded by the government as its own responsibility in wartime, a nationally planned and financed service, based on regional groups of hospitals, was accepted as the only satisfactory solution.

With the formation of the emergency hospital scheme, new areas of tension were added to those already in existence. In theory, at least, there were now two hospital services in England and Wales superimposed on two hospital systems: one service for special wartime purposes and another for the ordinary sick. One was nationally directed and financed; the other was not. The same doctors and nurses worked sometimes in one, and sometimes in the other. The dividing line ran right through the individual hospital. Strong and repeated efforts were made to keep it in sight, but often it was blurred and occasionally it was invisible.

The Health Departments soon found that they could not limit their interests and activities to the emergency sector of the hospital services as they had originally intended. Government responsibility was expanding in nearly every branch of social provision, and hospital work could not continue to be unaffected by the general trend of social development.

The assumption by the central authorities of these new responsibilities was at the same time stimulated by the progress and achievements of the emergency hospital scheme. Developments in one branch of the hospital services could not fail to influence those in another. Both war victims and sick civilians needed hospital attention and it was in the public interest that they should get it. But the hospital resources of the country were not large enough for this double task, and they were not, moreover, always used to the best advantage. All through the war, painful issues of priority arose which could not be settled at the centre. There was no authority in a position to tackle the problem of hospital needs as a whole. The means and the powers of the Health Departments bore no relation to their greatly enlarged field of responsibility. As a result, the price paid by the civilian sick for the achievements of the emergency hospital scheme was larger than it would otherwise have been.

The price was increased, too, by the conditions of strain and shortage in which the hospitals had to do their work. The armed forces inevitably had prior claims on doctors, nurses and other hospital staffs, and the war industries absorbed many of the domestic workers. The nursing problem, already present before the war, became more acute as demands increased, thus forcing the government to concern itself with questions of recruiting, distributing and keeping nurses in hospitals. As regards the supply of doctors, the position was that, in the later years of the war, most of those who still staffed the civilian hospitals (apart from the newly qualified and inexperienced) were the elderly and the unfit. Many of these doctors, and nurses too, had to carry a heavy load of responsibility when, in more normal times and by virtue of their age, their burdens would have been eased. The price for the success of the emergency medical service was, therefore, partly paid by the hospital staffs themselves in terms of long hours of work and crowded hospitals under the strains of war and bombing. In all other respects the social costs fell upon the civilian patients, men, women and children, who stood at the end of the queue for hospital beds. Part of this cost was carried over into the post-war years.

The emergency medical service should not, however, be judged solely on its achievements in action and the costs it entailed. It left behind a heritage of advances in hospital care, and a fund of knowledge and experience in organisation and administration. It demonstrated, in its limited field, what a hospital service could be, and it gave many institutions of varying character and type their first real opportunity to work together for a common purpose. This was not the result of deliberate acts of policy. History was often made by seemingly insignificant and unconnected decisions imposed by immediate necessities and carried out despite formidable psychological and practical handicaps. The demands of war were inescapable, but once accepted, they produced ideas as relevant to the needs of peace as of war.

It was only two years after the outbreak of war – and just when a second winter of air bombardment was expected – that the Minister of Health and the Secretary of State for Scotland made their statement about the future of Britain's hospital services. "It is the objective of the Government, as soon as may be after war, to ensure that by means of a comprehensive hospital service appropriate treatment shall be readily available to every person in need of it" (Hansard, 9 October 1941, vol 374, col 1116). At that time, no fundamental changes in the ownership and finance of hospitals were contemplated, but it was announced that hospital surveys would be started immediately "to provide the information needed as a basis for future plans". By 1946, when the last results of the surveys had been published, more was known about Britain's hospital resources and needs than had ever been known before. This was the first step on the road towards reconstruction.

The policy background

My task is to explore the relations between thought and action in the field of health legislation since the appearance in 1905 of Dicey's *Law and opinion in England in the nineteenth century.*

What I have chosen to examine, expressed at its simplest, is the organisation of medical care within the social and scientific context of the last 50 years [the first half of the 20th century]. What forces have shaped those institutions and systems, public and private, individual and collective, through which doctor and patient are brought together? There have, of course, been many; health is a relative concept, deeply embedded, as a doctor has said, "in the domains of politics, philosophy, etiquette, religion, cosmology and kinship" (Paul, 1955, p 459). All I have attempted in this paper is to single out a few of the principal strands of influence on thought and action in the 20th century.

The National Health Insurance Act of 1911 and the National Health Service Act of 1946 summarise the two great periods of legislative activity in the provision of personal health services in England. During both periods, the figure of a Welshman galvanised BMA House [home of the British Medical Association] into action. The decisions of these two men, the counsellors they chose and the bargains they struck have profoundly affected the structure of our health institutions and the place of the doctor in modern England.

Accordingly, this paper concentrates attention on the events of 1911 and 1946. First, I shall discuss some of the difficulties of disentangling the current of social forces and opinion from the influence of war on policies for health. Second, I describe the conditions of general practice before the Act of 1911 – the general practitioner's Act. Third, I attempt to trace the impact of science on medicine as one of the forces which contributed to the Act of 1946 – the specialist's Act. Binding these topics together, I employ a common political thread. In a sentence, it is the unreality of the antithesis between 'collectivism' and 'individualism' in the problem of the clash between equality and freedom.

This was one of the problems which dominated the debates about health and social policy at the beginning of the 20th century. In framing the Act of 1911, Lloyd George, as he impishly remarked, renounced vice, in the person of Beatrice Webb with her scheme for a public salaried medical service, and virtuously embraced insurance (Bunbury and Titmuss, 1957). She turned out to be the lady from the Pru; courted and introduced by a rising young solicitor in the insurance world, later to become Chancellor of the Exchequer, Sir

Kingsley Wood. Although of respectable actuarial parentage, she had an uncommonly high record of lapses. These, however, she successfully concealed and got herself 'approved' as a friendly body, cheerfully able to dispense on the doorsteps of the poor both health and burial benefits. Thus fortified, Lloyd George was able to provide working-class breadwinners with medical benefits and free choice of doctor. In 1946, Aneurin Bevan climbed on to Lloyd George's shoulders and gave to the middle classes and to women and children what the working man had received in 1911. Not only did Bevan renounce vice, on this occasion represented by the coalition government's plan for a salaried medical service controlled by local government, but he also renounced Miss Prudential, leaving her to be cultivated by Lord Beveridge and a new generation of pension consultants and retirement counsellors.

The question that is often asked by students from abroad of comparative social policies is why has state intervention in the field of medical care in England advanced further than in any other country in the Western world. Part of the answer is that the 1946 legislation would have assumed a very different and less comprehensive form but for the fact of 1911, and but for the fact that it happened when it did – paradoxically, so close in time and in thought to the philosophy of individualism. We are thus led to examine the social and economic problems of medical care during the first decade of the century.

In the introduction to the second edition of his book, written in 1914, Dicey (1926, 2nd edn, p 74) sagaciously remarked: "A collectivist never holds a stronger position than when he advocates the enforcement of the best ascertained laws of health". For the state to act in the interests of "the best ascertained laws of health", meant, to him, a grave threat to liberty, for such action signified "government for the good of the people by experts, or officials who know, or think they know, what is good for the people better than either any non-official person or than the mass of the people themselves" (ibid, p 73). This was collectivism or socialism; Dicey used both terms as synonyms, although he preferred the former because it was a convenient antithesis to individualism. In any event, the motive behind the law and the effect of the law itself signified to Dicey more redistributive taxation in favour of the poor. He assumed that all state intervention in the field of health had this consequence.

Both theses – that more enforcement of the laws of health means more collectivism and less personal liberty, and that such measures benefit only the poor – may be examined in the light of other ideas and forces which Dicey neglected.

He conceived of opinion as "law-making opinion" that "body of beliefs, convictions, sentiments, accepted principles, or firmly rooted prejudices" which, taken together, makes up the "tone of England" at a particular time (ibid, p 73). I must stray from this conception.

Although Dicey, at the time he wrote, may justly be absolved from neglecting Freud, no one who attempts to trace the course of ideas and action in the field of health over the the first half of the 20th century can fail to note the impress of a growing body of psychological and psychoanalytical knowledge. New knowledge has put health and disease in a new cultural perspective. Personal illness has acquired a social definition. Psychiatry and society may now confirm the patient's subjective definition of illness. The patient, as Péquignot (1954) has said, has once again to be listened to.

Advances in knowledge in other scientific fields have also had a profound influence on law and opinion about health; about what Sherrington (1955), the biologist, called "the urge-to-live". I think of the influence on medical opinion, if not on lay opinion, even when Dicey was writing, of Darwin and Galton, Virchow and Pasteur, Koch and Ehrlich, Gowland Hopkins and others. By the beginning of the 20th century, the new scientific era in medicine was well under way. Nevertheless, Dicey found no place in his survey of opinion for the influence of these and other developments in the natural sciences. By 1905, they were important for at least three reasons: diagnosis now began to matter more as the empirical role of expectant treatment, of folk therapeutics, waned in the face of the advances of rational medicine; specialisation in knowledge and skill was developing rapidly, thus affecting the organisation of medical service, the structure of the profession, accepted norms of ethical behaviour, and the doctor–patient relationship; lastly, the costs of medical care to the individual were beginning to rise, the first warning of the coming technological revolution.

These movements – scientific, professional and economic – were shifting the emphasis, in matters of health and disease, from the situation to the person; from the environment to the individual; from the public health officer to the general practitioner. Scientific intervention from without and changes in medical training within were altering the pattern of practice. Together, they produced the professional concept of the general practitioner. He had not existed before as a separate, distinctive branch of the medical profession with a set of recognisable roles and functions. He had to be created to enable the new medicine at the end of the century to be practised. But this was not enough. What was also needed were systems and institutions which would allow and, indeed, encourage the doctors to practise as they wanted to practise. In what they wanted to do and be, they were, of course, influenced by the changing expectations placed on them by the 'new' medicine of the times. Basically, it was a problem of social organisation. The natural sciences were responsible for making it a social problem.

Simultaneously, developments in the comparative method of studying society, statistical and sociological, were helping England to identify its problems of health and disease more precisely and more historically (there now being available a more adequate body of knowledge for estimating trends over time). The concept of progress, of improvement or the lack of it, came to be applied in more sophisticated ways to the national health. Population groups, their social, occupational and class characteristics, increasingly became the material for epidemiological studies of disease and death. What had been in the forefront of medical thought and action half a century earlier was 'the health of towns'. By the beginning of the 20th century, the emerging problem of ascertaining the 'best laws of health' was the health of individuals in their social setting, especially the health of mothers and children. Society was beginning to count and reassess the health costs of industrial progress in terms of the life chances of its next generation of workers, mothers and soldiers.

Significantly, the century was ushered in with a Midwives Act, and the health, nutrition and medical care of mothers and babies, schoolchildren and military recruits became a respectable, even a popular, subject of parliamentary debate. No longer could it be said, with Bagehot, that "the character of the poor is an unfit topic for continuous art". War as a measure of national, even imperial, stamina, exploded the doctrine of 'natural justice', confounded the works on political economy which, as Bagehot remarked, always began with the supposition of two men cast on an uninhabited island, and stimulated a burst of medical inquiries and legislative activity concerning the ills of the working classes.

The prolonged social inquest that followed the Boer War showed that little comfort could be drawn from the study of historical trends in mortality rates as indicators of levels of health. Three quarters of a century of industrial and sanitary progress, of accumulating wealth and the acquisition of an Empire, had had no obvious effect, for example, on the infant death rate (Logan, 1950). It was as high at the beginning of the 20th century as it had been in the 1840s; higher than it was to be, 50 years later, in most of the 'under-developed' areas of the world. Considered in this biological context, England, at the turn of the 20th century, was falling behind the rest of Western society in its care of the young. In 1902, the Inspector-General of Army Recruiting spoke gloomily of "the gradual deterioration of the physique of the working-classes from whom the bulk of the recruits must always be drawn" (Ministry of Defence, 1904). Whatever its moral implications, here was a clear warning. Society was giving insufficient thought to investment in the next generation. Material thrift was not enough.

What emerged from all this debate about our military fortunes and our standards of communal fitness was a new accent on prevention; a redefinition of the idea in personal terms – the prevention of premature death, sickness and ill-health; the 'seeds of decay' among the young. But to accept this redefinition of prevention and advocate its endorsement meant, however, a challenge to prevailing social values in at least two respects. It meant enlarging the area of social responsibility – attaching more responsibility to someone, some group, some authority – and it also meant practical action.

As knowledge increased of the causal factors in disease and as advances in the natural sciences began to penetrate the practice of medicine, it became clearer that action meant social action and responsibility collective responsibility. The logic of knowledge and an increasing public awareness of the potentialities of action based on advances in knowledge, revealed the limits within which individuals could determine their own health. The expert (disliked by Dicey) knew better. Supported by science, by the need for forethought and prediction, by the demand for national wellbeing, by the idea of progress, the potential power of technical medicine increased. The story of medicine in society over the ensuing 50 years is, in general, a story of the accelerating force of these ideas and trends – a process dramatically hastened by two world wars and the scientific discovery of malnutrition during the 1930s.

During the first decade of the 20th century, however, the organised structure of applied medicine was in no condition to absorb and practise either the 'scientific triumphs of the laboratory' or the idea of prevention. The advance of these conflicting yet complementary forces, the scientific and the social, was hindered by a variety of barriers: economic, professional and institutional. Changes were needed, for instance, in the economic structure within which most doctors practised, if the benefits of these advances in knowledge were to be reaped in terms of an improvement in the quality of medical care. The general practitioner was the key figure in this problem of change. Then, as now [1958], hospital provision, public and voluntary, catered for only a tiny proportion of the total expressed demand for medical attention. The provision of medical care for the mass of the people centred round the general practitioners: their training, their conditions of work, and their relationships with their patients and fellow doctors. The intervention of the state in the field of medical care in 1911, and to a greater degree in 1948, cannot be fully understood unless account is taken of the situation of general practice prior to the rise of 'socialised' medicine. The opinion of the doctor, particularly the rank-and-file doctor, was a powerful force in shaping the future course of the law in relation to health.

Before the Act of 1911, the working lives and material standards of the majority of general practitioners were profoundly affected by their relationships not only with the administrators of the Poor Law but also with a network of long-established social institutions. These took many forms, for their primary functions were not to provide medical care. Most of them were voluntary and philanthropic associations; friendly society clubs, trade union clubs, slate clubs, works clubs, tontines, breaking societies, charitable dispensaries, and so forth. Then there were the medical aid societies run on private enterprise lines by insurance companies. The dominant system of medical care, organised through this complex of institutions and groups, was known as 'contract medical practice' (British Medical Association, 1905). The doctor was the 'club' or group doctor; for a stated sum of money per week or per year (generally a capitation fee), the doctor contracted to provide professional service (and in many cases medicine) for the members of the group.

The mass of the wage-earning population, small shopkeepers and a substantial proportion of the middle classes received their medical care through this system of contract practice. Generally there was no maximum wage or salary limit, although the doctors strongly opposed the inclusion of middle-class members, partly because they made greater demands on their services than the working classes. Consequently, they criticised, although without much success, the system of fixing contributions, in each individual club, on a flat-rate basis. In the opinion of the doctors a few years later, one of the signal gains made by the profession from the 1911 legislation was the exclusion of the middle classes not only from the benefits of state insurance but also from contract practice. With the withdrawal of the working classes, club and contract practice virtually collapsed after 1911. It could no longer be sustained without the contributions of the workers.

Before this happened, however, contract practice, expressly developed for wage and salary earners, generally excluded wives and other dependants, the old, the disabled and other 'bad' risks. It was a system of medical care for men at work, regularly at work. Then, as now, the actuarial bad risks were not courted by any insurance system, voluntary or commercial, of prepaid medical care. All these excluded classes thus had to seek their medical care elsewhere, mainly from out-patient departments, 'sixpenny doctors' and the Poor Law. In so far as they were treated, they generally saw a different doctor. Thus, for the mass of the population, 'family doctoring' did not exist. Perhaps 10% to 20% of families had a private, 'fee-for-service' doctor for the whole family (Money Chiozza, 1912). The term 'family doctor' was not then in use. It does not figure, for instance, in the 96-page report by the British Medical Association in 1905 on *Contract practice*. Its gradual acceptance later in the century, as a principle of more effective medical care, grew out of the concept of prevention.

This period of transition from the folk medicine of the 19th century to rational medicine in the 20th century was characterised by a widespread revolt among the doctors against the developing system of contract practice. Culminating in the legislation of 1911, this period can be seen as one in which the doctors were engaged in a

Hobbesian struggle for independence from the power and authority exercised over their lives, their work and their professional values by voluntary associations and private enterprise. The 'Battle of the Clubs', as it was called, was, fundamentally, a struggle for professional and private freedom. Scientific developments in medicine, the emergence of a stronger hierarchical structure based on more specialisation in knowledge and skill, and new ideas about health and disease called for radical changes in the ways in which doctor and patient were brought together. One change that was needed was an enlargement of professional freedom.

Although, as a professional group, they are by no means alone in this respect, doctors have, at various times since at least the beginning of the 20th century, shown a marked dislike for organisation; for administrators; for bureaucrats – especially local bureaucrats and bourgeois councillors. They showed this dislike, for instance, during the negotiations with the government before the introduction of the Health Service. It was then made clear that in no circumstances whatever would the profession entertain the idea of local government having any responsibility for the hospital and general medical services (Eckstein, 1955). The present structure of the Health Service owes more to the opinion of doctors than to political and public opinion.

Medical hostility to lay organisations was fomented and sharpened before the Act of 1911. We may briefly consider some of the forces which helped to strengthen this powerful heritage.

First, there was the issue of professional independence and clinical freedom. Under these contract systems of medical care, doctors had no security of tenure. They could be dismissed at any time. They were forced to compete and tender for these appointments. There was no free choice in the doctor–patient relationship. As they were always liable to be reported to an 'impertinent' lay committee for inattention, they felt unable to resist demands from patients for medicine (British Medical Association, 1905). They had no right of appeal under the 'administrative law' of these voluntary associations. As full-time salaried doctors, they were often "unmercifully sweated" by insurance companies (Little, 1932, p 201) at rates of pay; they were under pressure to sign certificates and life assurance forms against their medical judgement, and they were expected to canvass for new patients. In short, the power over their professional lives exercised by these voluntary associations and private concerns was felt by the majority of general practitioners as an intolerable infringement on their liberty to practise medicine. The system of medical care under the Poor Law had similar degrading effects on the large number of doctors who undertook these part-time appointments (Webb and Webb, 1910).

Second, the doctors complained of the demoralising influence on their work and their patients of many patent and proprietary medicines: the 'secret remedies' as they were called, courageously attacked for a decade or more by the British Medical Association. Out of a total estimated expenditure of £12 million on all drugs, dressings and appliances in 1907, over one quarter (£3.25 million) was spent on these 'secret remedies' which claimed to cure every conceivable disease (Prest and Adams, 1954, p 157). For most newspapers, the advertising of these drugs (on which £2 million was annually spent) constituted a major source of income. Newspaper proprietors (later to oppose the National Health Insurance Bill with unexampled violence) played no small part in the formation of opinion on maters of health and disease.

An incredulous public, dazzled by the new scientific jargon, misled by doctors who cut their ethical corners, confused by Chambers of Commerce who defended these 'secret remedies' in the name of freedom of contract, exploited by the entire press of the country, became, as one critic said, 'permanent medicine swallowers'. The average doctor's sense of powerlessness under contract practice was accentuated by this traffic in drugs. As a scientific revolution in medicine developed, the 'bottle of medicine habit' became more deeply embedded in the culture of health and disease (British Medical Association, 1909).

Third, the doctors complained bitterly about their standard of living. Beatrice and Sidney Webb (1910, p 253) concluded their survey in 1910: "... the medical profession in the United Kingdom stands at this moment in a position of grave danger. A very large proportion of its members earn incomes which can only be described as scandalously inadequate, whilst many of those who now enter its ranks after a long and expensive education fail altogether to secure a footing". It is doubtful whether many general practitioners were the products of public schools; certainly not as high a proportion as now enter the teaching hospitals (Kelsall, 1957).

Low standards of living, combined with the competitive practices of voluntary associations, philanthropic institutions and commercial insurance companies, led to widespread abuses. The medical journals of the period resound with the cries of doctor against doctor about the bribery and corruption, the employment of unqualified assistants, the fee-splitting, the canvassing, the underselling and commission-taking that was apparently widespread. As a body, general practitioners campaigned against the voluntary hospitals for giving the middle classes cheap out-patient treatment; against the rising generation of specialist surgeons and consultants for reducing the standard of living of general practitioners; and against the clubs for allowing the middle classes to obtain medical care at the same capitation fee as the working classes. In its values and goals, the profession was divided against itself; a reflection, in some senses, of the increasing division of labour within medicine. In this situation, more power fell into the hands of the organisation men of the times: the administrators, lay committees and bureaucrats of the voluntary associations and insurance companies. "The cause of these evils", concluded the British Medical Association report (1905, p 28), "is the advantage which non-medical organizations are able to take of the competition between individual medical practitioners".

In February 1910 (before Lloyd George had introduced his Health Insurance Bill), the *British Medical Journal* (editorial, 1910, vol 1, pp 521 and 713) wrote: "We are thus reduced to a dilemma from which most people see no escape except by some form ... of State assistance". It went on, in this and succeeding editorials, to offer to collaborate with the government in a state scheme provided that no lay committee or "sham philanthropy" came between the profession and the government.

The rest of this story of how the foundations of the National Health Service were laid is better known (Bunbury and Titmuss, 1957). In the battle over the 1911 legislation, the doctors forced Lloyd George to give them satisfaction on most of their important claims: control of medical benefit not by friendly societies and clubs, but by special 'insurance committees' on which doctors would be represented; freedom of choice; the right of every doctor to take part in the service; security of tenure, the exclusion of the middle classes and higher capitation fees. Compared with what had obtained before, the material rewards for most general practitioners were approximately doubled. Years later, the British Medical Association's official historian had no doubt that the position of the profession had been "vastly improved" (Little, 1932, p 328). In terms of professional service, the law of 1911 provided more opportunity for the better expression of the ethical code of medical practice; corruption and competition could diminish; and, for a large section of doctors and patients alike, freedom of choice became a more genuine possibility.

This is my interpretation of the health law of 1911 and the ideas and movements that helped to shape it. To Dicey (1926 edn, pp 33 and 53), it "vehemently expressed the growth of collectivism" for the benefit of the working classes or "the pampered classes", as *The Times* described them (10 June 1911). The fundamental issue in 1911 was not, I suggest, between individualism and collectivism, between contract and status; but between different forms of collectivism, different degrees of freedom; open or concealed power. To whom should the doctor be accountable in society? How was scientific progress to be incorporated into the practice of medicine? What, in the light of advancing physical and psychological knowledge, were 'the best ascertained laws of health'?

I must now move on from 1911. In retrospect, it represents one of the great dividing periods in the development of systems of medical care. It happened when it did because of the conjunction of many historical forces. The power of private contract practice was perhaps the most important single factor. Its origins are clearly traceable to the social conditions created by industrialisation. It grew to power in the vacuum left by individualism. By the turn of the 20th century, there had developed what might be called a 'coalition of interests' between the needs of the doctors to incorporate new knowledge in their practices and to pursue their calling in accordance with the ethics sanctioned by their group, and the needs of the working population to conserve their health and wage-earning power from all the hazards of industrial and technological change. Both were conscious of the power exercised over their lives by these different external forces. Thus, the Act of 1911 had more to do with professional liberty than with class warfare; more with freedom of contract than with equalitarian redistribution.

By 1946, the fundamental issues were in some senses the same, in other senses different. The emphasis shifted to the social rights of all citizens to better health. By then, science had become a much more potent force in the problems facing modern society of choosing between alternative systems of medical care. Not only was medicine more powerful, but more had been learnt about the inequalities of health and medical care between different social classes and occupations. Studies of infant mortality by social class had shown, for example, that, despite the great absolute decline among all classes, the relative gap between the highest and the lowest rates was, if anything, somewhat greater in 1950 than in 1911 (Morris and Heady, 1955). Elsewhere, evidence was growing that the rich were benefiting more and earlier than the poor from advances in scientific knowledge. The most striking instance here is the long period that elapsed, after the early 1920s, before the working classes drew anything like a proportionate benefit from the discovery of insulin for the treatment of the young insulin-sensitive diabetic (Morris, 1957, p 27).

As more recognition was accorded to the social factors in health and disease, it became clearer that the quality and distribution of medical care was one of the central issues for social policy. The advent of scientific medicine made it clearer still.

During the period between these two health laws of 1911 and 1946, science was invading medicine at an accelerating pace. After the discovery of prontosil in 1935, the process became more marked and challenging. Once the medical significance of new knowledge in the biological and natural sciences has been grasped, the floodgates between theory and practice in medical care burst wide open. Developments now read like a story of geometrical progression: they include the elaboration of penicillin, streptomycin, oleandomycin and other antibiotics; the application of nuclear physics; improvements in anaesthesia and anti-coagulants; knowledge of blood compatibility; and the discovery of cortisone and polio vaccines.

The advent of rational medicine and developments in psychological knowledge have led to the growth of the idea in Western society that pain is avoidable by rational, non-mystical means. As standards of education and living rise, greater significance is attached to sensations of pain as signals of danger to individuals and their sense of self-preservation. An American study of "cultural components in responses to pain" has shown that the educational background of the patients plays an important role in their attitude to the symptomatic meaning of pain sensation. "The more educated patients are more health-conscious and more aware of pain as a possible symptom of a dangerous disease" (Zborowski, 1952, p 27).

The support that middle-class opinion in England has given to the NHS and the nature of the demands that these classes have made upon it become explicable in the context of ideas and expectations of this kind. What has been learnt from a variety of medical and sociological studies suggests that the middle classes are more conscious of the need for health as an essential element in achieving 'success in life'; more aware of the technical and psychological potentialities in medicine; readier to see, as Clark-Kennedy (1957, p 87) has said, that the power of medicine over individual lives "has increased, is increasing and is likely to increase still further", and, above all, quicker to recognise that the costs to the individual of medical care have been pushed to unprecedented heights by a technological revolution.

For the Labour government, in 1946, to have simply extended the old Health Insurance Scheme to include wives and dependants and hospital benefits would have meant excluding the middle classes. From a working-class standpoint, this could well have been interpreted as a perpetuation of the pre-war system of two standards of medical care: 'panel' and private. In practice, however, the likelihood is that the position of the classes would have been reversed. The 'protected' working classes would have been, relatively speaking, the largest beneficiaries of scientific medicine. The middle classes, fully exposed in a private market to the initial inflationary phase of technical change, would have suffered. Technical progress would have behaved towards them as the gods behaved towards Tantalus.

This, however, was not one of the decisive arguments in 1945, but many of the consultants (represented by the Royal Colleges) did see the writing on the professional wall. They foresaw the coming bankruptcy of the voluntary hospitals; the threat (to the profession) of greater local government control; the harmful financial effects on doctors as well as patients of the rise in the private costs of health; and the dominant role to be played in the future by the hospital – and especially the teaching hospital – as it increasingly became the focus of medical science and technology, the laboratory for "the Golden Age of surgery" (Wakeley, 1957), and the main source of prestige and power. With shrewdness and foresight, the Royal Colleges led the medical profession into the NHS and helped to shape a law which made available the benefits of scientific medicine to all classes in the community.

But this, I believe, would not have come about but for the Second World War and the Labour government. The first supplied the decisive motive-power, the second the will. One of the lessons of the war, as a citizens' war, was the popular demand for the abolition of the Poor Law; of ineligible citizens; of personally merited disease; of inequality before 'the best ascertained laws of health'. The National Health Service Act of 1946 was, in part, an expression of this wartime mood for justice and equality of opportunity. But, in a longer perspective of time and social change, it was a renewal of the argument for the freedom of patients and doctors. Once again, although in circumstances dramatically altered by technical progress, the choice was between different forms of collectivism and a different distribution of power between the doctor and the administrator, and between the representatives of the people and the profession.

There are some who still see the Act as a collectivist device for the sole benefit of the working classes. As the offspring of 1911, it is depicted as the apex of 'welfare state' benevolence. But this is too simple, as it was too simple a view of 1911. Of course the working classes have benefited, but the middle classes have benefited even more, and the medical profession most of all (Cox, 1950). The economic and financial effects of state intervention in the sphere of health and disease since 1946 are complex and, I have no doubt, have worked out differently from the often accepted views of what 'welfare statism' is thought to mean in practice.

Although the demand for social justice has been one of the major forces shaping law and opinion in the field of health since the beginning of the 20th century, other forces have played an equal – and sometimes, more important – role. One, as I have shown, is the advancement of scientific knowledge. Another is represented by the movement from fatalism to awareness in popular attitudes towards health and disease. Yet another is the recurrent business of liberal thought to release the individual (whether, in this context, doctor or patient) from unalterable dependence on any particular social group. In short, the underlying aim of health legislation has been to prevent social injustice by countering power with power. The law of 1946 was directed towards the diffusion of power, the diffusion of the power of medicine and the diffusion of the benefits of science. These were its aims; what has happened in reality is inevitably another story.

The structure of the NHS in England

De Tocqueville, opening a chapter on 'The desire for wealth' in his famous treatise on *Democracy in America* (1946, p 398) wrote: "In America the passion for physical wellbeing ... is general". He saw this passion for bodily comfort, for a sense of individual ease, as an inseparable part of a desire for material wellbeing.

Today [1957], one might venture to say that Americans want to be healthy, physically and psychologically, because they are constantly aware of a need to be healthy. This consciousness of need, its degree of intensity, and the forms of behaviour in which it finds expression, is in large measure the product of the cultural forces which play on the individual from childhood to old age. What society expects of individuals and, reciprocally, what individuals themselves feel is expected of them by their fellows, thus represent, in the effects they have in conditioning attitudes to health, important variables in the demand for medical care. Good health is seen both as a pre-requisite for the success of the personality and, simultaneously, as a necessary condition for the enjoyment and exploitation of success.

In general terms, it can thus be argued that, the larger the investment by any society in 'individualism' (as a 'way of life'), the more may 'health-consciousness' spread. Similarly, the limits to what is personally conceived to be tolerable in feelings of bad health or inadequate function may also rise. And, as society becomes more health-conscious (in the sense of more individuals becoming aware of the higher standards expected of them), the more may each individual become dependent, or at least feel dependent, in an age of scientific medicine, on other individuals – on resources external to themselves for the achievement of good health. The high esteem of psychology and science in the American culture both emphasises and expresses this sense of dependency in the search for good health.

In relative terms, individuals may come to feel more dependent on psychotherapy, on medical science, on the doctors; less on their own inner resources. The high prestige accorded today to the physician is not, therefore, in this context surprising. Nor, perhaps, should we be surprised by the particular roles pursued by the collectivity of doctors – the American Medical Association. They are the organised and centralised reflections of ascribed power – the power ascribed by society as a whole to those who are regarded as professional experts in matters of health and disease, life and death. Within limits, each distinctive culture gets the medical priesthood it wants.

It is, however, one thing for society to agree on the importance of good health and good medical care; quite another for it to agree on how good health may be achieved and maintained by organising and distributing its medical resources in alternative ways. I shall, therefore, take as my main theme the organisation of medical care, and shall discuss some of the important issues raised by the introduction in 1948 of a National Health Service (NHS) in England and Wales.

* * * * *

The legal foundation of the NHS is the Act passed by Parliament in 1946. The service began to operate in July 1948. Subsequent legislative measures and ministerial regulations issued under the authority of the principal Act have also to be taken into account in considering the present administrative framework.

At the head is the Minister of Health, advised by the Central Health Services Council and a number of Standing Advisory Committees. These are chiefly composed of professional people, representative of the various interests, who are appointed by the Minister after consultation with the organisations concerned. In practice, the Minister appoints those who are nominated by the professions.

It is the Minister's duty, in the words of the 1946 Act, "to promote the establishment in England and Wales of a comprehensive health service designed to secure improvement in the physical and mental health of the people of England and Wales and the prevention, diagnosis and treatment of illness, and for that purpose to provide or secure the effective provision of services". It is further laid down, "The services so provided shall be free of charge, except where any provision of this Act expressly provides for the making and recovery of charges".

Any general impression that the NHS is entirely a 'free' service (in the sense of being free on demand) requires correction.

The principle of free access to medical care, a fundamental principle in the development of the NHS in 1948, has to some extent been limited in recent years [early 1950s], primarily in respect of dental and ophthalmic care. Some limitation to the effective use of the NHS has been brought about as a result of the fall in the relative value of sickness benefits under the National Insurance Scheme. At the end of 1956, these benefits represented only about 34% of average industrial earnings for a man, wife and two children (*Ministry of Labour Gazette*, September 1957). Some workers may be unwilling to consult their doctors; others may be compelled to return to work too soon.

An essential element in the principle of free access to medical care is freedom to use or not to use the NHS, and to choose and change one's doctor. Today, some 550 to 600 general practitioners limit their work to private, fee-paying patients, and large numbers of other general practitioners combine NHS and private patient work. Patients can and do have an NHS general practitioner, pay privately for a consultant and use the free services of the NHS hospitals. Or they can pay a general practitioner and have access to free consultant and hospital services. Some have both a private and an NHS doctor (Gray and Cartwright, 1953, vol ii, p 1308).

The one limitation to this freedom of choice in the doctor–patient relationship that has been imposed since 1948 was forced on an unwilling Ministry of Health by the profession. In October 1950, restrictions were placed on the ease with which patients could change their doctors. The new arrangements led to some paperwork, introduced a waiting period before a change could be effective and, in most cases, required the written consent of the present doctor. Some patients have naturally found this an embarrassing procedure, as insured workers did in the 1930s when their liberties were restricted on the grounds that patients changed their doctors too frequently (Levy, 1944, p 117). Similar arguments were used after 1948 but, again, no evidence has been published to support these generalisations about 'excessive' changing of doctors. Among other patients today, with little knowledge about statutory regulations, an impression has gained ground that it is impossible or almost impossible to change one's doctor.

One theory held, it would seem, by younger practitioners, is that this restriction on freedom was insisted on by the British Medical Association in the interests of the older, well-established practitioners anxious to safeguard their practices in an era when the demands to enter medicine, including general practice, have been unprecedently high. In 1954, the government, responding to the anxieties of the profession, set up a committee (Committee to Consider the Future Number of Medical Practitioners), mainly composed of doctors, to consider whether Britain was not now training too many doctors.

* * * * *

Among all the ideas of the 1930s and 1940s which led to the creation of the NHS, the one which increasingly dominated the mind of the public and the profession alike was the idea of prevention: the prevention of ill-health and incapacity. In the field of medical care, the idea of prevention is largely a product of the 20th century, not because of any originality in the idea itself, but because of its recognised practicability. The impact of scientific advances on medicine enlarged the area and potentialities of preventive action; from the individual to the group, from the group to society. Above all, it raised the level of public expectation. I stress the significance here of the idea of prevention simply because of the important role it played in relation to the two fundamental principles on which the NHS came to be organised.

The first, in the words of the coalition government's White Paper of 1944, was "to divorce the care of health from questions of personal means or other factors irrelevant to it" (Ministry of Health, 1944, p 47). To those who stood by the principle of free access to medical care services by all who wanted to use them, it meant earlier and easier access to the doctor; thus enlarging the possibilities of preventive action. The acceptance of this principle meant "the creation of a new public responsibility; to make it in future somebody's clear duty to see that all medical facilities are available to all people....".

The method chosen to create this responsibility was to transfer to the new administrative bodies the existing voluntary and municipal hospitals with their clinics and other associated institutions. Some hospitals, nursing homes, institutions run by religious orders and certain facilities organised on a profit-making basis were not taken over. In all, the Minister of Health, with the government behind him and Parliament in ultimate control, became the nation's trustee for some 2,700 separate hospitals. Or, to put it in terms of the number of hospital beds, most of the remaining one fifth of beds not then in public ownership were transferred to the Minister (Guillebaud Committee, 1956, p 51). Many of them, and particularly the voluntary teaching hospitals, retained on their boards of governors and management committees a large number of people who had previously served them as voluntary institutions.

One alternative to common ownership was a contractual relationship with the voluntary hospitals. This method was eventually rejected.

There were weighty arguments in the debates which shaped the NHS in Britain. They took place during a phase of the war effort when the demand for the effective planning and organisation of the nation's resources was strong and widely expressed. Perhaps the most important argument in the planning approach was the need for 'territorial justice' - more equality of access to medical care services for people living in different parts of the country. In other words, a geographically comprehensive hospital service could not, it was thought, be provided under the aegis of some 2,000 separate, independent and often competing hospitals. There was no hospital system; this was the striking fact in a country as geographically small, densely populated and homogeneous as Britain. There was instead a collection of individual hospitals, criss-crossed, separated and enclosed by local government boundary barriers; legal, residential and occupational barriers; and medical category and financial barriers. There were, indeed, too many barriers to the 'right' kind of hospital, despite the fact that 80% of hospital beds were already provided as a public service. In the words of the government's White Paper (Ministry of Health, 1944, p 56): "The anomalies of large waiting lists in one hospital and suitable empty beds at another, and of the hospitals in the same area running duplicated specialist centres which could be better concentrated in one more highly equipped and staffed centre for the area, are largely the result of a situation in which hospital services are many people's business but nobody's full responsibility".

Attempts, during the preceding 20 years, in a few local areas to coordinate policy and administration among voluntary and public hospitals had, with one or two exceptions, failed completely (Sankey Committee, 1937). This was no theoretical surmise; it was borne out by the experience gained in the organisation of the wartime Emergency Hospital Scheme based on regional hospital areas (Titmuss, 1950). These were the lessons of history which led, in 1948, to the creation of new administrative and executive instruments. These new instruments, regional hospital boards and local hospital management committees, represented the one major administrative innovation of the Health Service Act. For the organisation and administration of the rest of the personal health services, the Act drew on the past.

* * * * *

Now that the NHS has been in operation for about nine years [1948–57], can any conclusions be drawn about this experiment in 'socialised medicine'? How has it worked in practice? Has it led to a deterioration in standards of medical care? What effect has it had on the doctor–patient relationship? Has the removal of the financial barrier unleashed a great demand; led to much abuse of general practitioners' time; converted them into signers of certificates, sorters of minor maladies and hospital referral agents? What effect has the NHS had on the profession itself; on levels of remuneration, career prospects, clinical freedom and the position of doctors in the power structure of administration? Lastly, but by no means exhaustively, is it true that the costs of the NHS have risen so steeply that it is in danger of getting out of control?

I thus come to a brief summary of the Guillebaud Report (1956) which, in many ways, stands as a landmark in the history of the NHS. Its publication marked a stage when the initial and, to a large extent, transitory, problems had been mainly overcome. The dimensions of the more fundamental and long-term issues in the organisation of medical care are now in clearer perspective.

This report was the product of a five-member committee of inquiry set up by the government in May 1953 under the chairmanship of a distinguished Cambridge economist. Its terms of reference were: "To review the present and prospective cost of the National Health Service; to suggest means, whether by modifications in organization or otherwise, of ensuring the most effective control and efficient use of such Exchequer funds as may be made available; to advise how, in view of the burdens on the Exchequer, a rising charge upon it can be avoided while providing for the maintenance of an adequate Service; and to make recommendations".

The Committee was set up at a time when a powerful body of opinion in the country held the view that this public enterprise was failing. Costs were getting out of control, or, as the *British Medical Journal* (Editorial, 2 December 1950) put it: "The National Health Service is heading for the bankruptcy court . . . and we are facing bankruptcy because of the Utopian finances of the Welfare State". Another major criticism was that the administrative structure of the NHS had too many defects: it was over-centralised; it had curtailed the professional freedom of the doctor; it had given the administrator and the lay member too much power; and the division of functions under different authorities was having unfortunate effects on both doctor and patient.

Soon after it was set up, the Committee asked the National Institute of Economic and Social Research (a private institute distinguished for its contributions to economic research) to undertake a detailed analysis of the costs of the NHS. The task was entrusted to Brian Abel-Smith and myself. The main part of the memorandum on costs we submitted, which was accepted by the Committee, was published in its report. The whole of our study was simultaneously published as a book (Abel-Smith and Titmuss, 1956).

In the words of the report, "The rising cost of the Service in real terms during the years 1948-54 was kept within narrow bounds.... Any charge that there has been widespread extravagance in the Service, whether in respect of the spending of money or the use of manpower, is not borne out by our evidence". The cost per head of the population at constant prices was, in fact, almost the same in 1953-54 as in 1949-50 (the first full year of operation). Moreover, the proportion of total national resources (the gross national product) paid for by public authorities fell from 3.75% in 1949-50 to 3.25% in 1953-54. All the estimates I have seen of the proportion of national resources devoted to medical care in the US give higher figures (but include private expenditure) and also show that the cost per head of the population has risen significantly since 1948.

These conclusions about the cost of the NHS came as a surprise to public opinion. What was expected was a strong recommendation for economy; for restriction; for more charges on patients. Instead, there were recommendations for spending (especially capital expenditure on hospitals and welfare provisions for older people) and for the reduction or removal of certain existing charges. One can only conclude that, for nearly seven years, public opinion both in England and the US had been seriously misled, partly because of the inadequate way in which public accounts are presented, partly because of a too simple faith in the validity of official statistics (particularly of estimates made during the war of what the new service might cost), and partly because powerful sections of medical and lay opinion were committed too soon to the view that the costs of 'socialised medicine' were bound to be astronomical.

In interpreting this conclusion that the cost of the NHS has been kept within narrow limits, the following summarised facts should be borne in mind: in proportion to the populations at risk, over this period, the hospitals did more work both in-patient and out-patient; more doctors (especially consultants), nurses, social workers, administrators, physiotherapists and other professional staffs, later to engage in private practice or other employment at home or abroad, were trained at public expense; more confinements took place in hospital; more road accidents were treated; more provision was made for industrial accidents which would otherwise have called for an expansion of health services organised by employers; a great increase took place in the use of X-rays, pathological and diagnostic services; more of these services were made directly available to general practitioners (in part a switch from the doctor's private practice expenses to the hospital service); the number of voluntary blood donations rose dramatically by over 300,000 to 760,000 in 1955 (*British Medical Journal*, 1956, ii, p 128); a larger proportion of those in need were fitted with hearing aids, artificial limbs, spectacles and dentures; more drug prescriptions were issued; more home helps and nursing services were provided for those who were ill at home; more doctors worked as NHS practitioners; there were fewer single-handed practitioners and more partnerships and group practices; the average number of people on a general practitioner's list fell; a substantial improvement took place in the geographical distribution of general practitioners and consultant services; finally, more medical research was undertaken and completed, as indicated by a striking rise in the flow of articles to scientific and medical journals after 1948.

Against this background of quantitative indices of performance, it is hardly surprising that the report found nothing basically unsound about the NHS's administrative structure. Taking account of the medical opposition to any form of local government control, it did not therefore propose any major changes in the existing tripartite structure. The report did, however, recommend, first, that steps should be taken to raise the quality of hospital administration (most of the existing staff were inherited from the old voluntary and municipal hospitals) and, second, that in the power structure of committees controlling the hospitals and general practitioner services, the proportion of medical membership should be reduced.

These are some of the more important findings of this investigation into the NHS. They hardly touch on the more subtle, intangible effects of the service on patient and doctor, nor on the critical questions of quality of medical care. They probably shed too comforting a glow on this experiment in public enterprise.

The NHS and general practice

There are a number of reasons which help to explain, even if they do not justify, the conclusion that the record of the health service is one of progress and success. Some of the more important ones become explicable only when it is understood how far-reaching were the effects of the Second World War [1939-45] on the British economy. The whole fabric of organised medical care, public and private, suffered particularly. Inevitably, the highest priorities in medicine were reserved for the military and civil defence forces. Even as early as June 1943, the standard of medical care available for the civilian population was, in the judgment of the War Cabinet, "dangerously low" (Titmuss, 1950, p 531). By the end of the war, the ranks of the general practitioners had been depleted by over one third; of those who remained, 10% were over 70 years of age, and in many industrial areas elderly doctors, educated before the First World War [1914-18] when general practice was little more than an empirical bedside art, were struggling with lists of 4,000 to 5,000 patients (Titmuss, 1950, p 530).

For over 15 years from 1939, no new hospital was built in Britain. Many of the voluntary hospitals which, by 1939, were virtually bankrupt and were only saved during the war by heavy government subsidies, faced, at the end of the war, an even more serious threat to their future (Titmuss, 1950, pp 450-8). Not only were these subsidies being withdrawn but the costs (and the standards expected) of medical care in hospital were rising on an unprecedented scale. The scientific revolution in medicine, beginning in the late 1930s, represented to most of the voluntary hospitals in Britain a sentence of death.

In the three years between the end of the war and the introduction of the NHS, when the air was thick with rumours about what was to happen to the hospitals, both the voluntary and municipal hospital authorities were unwilling to commit themselves to much expenditure. In some respects, therefore, hospital conditions deteriorated further.

When the service began to operate in 1948, it thus inherited the debts of a decade of sacrifice and neglect, financial poverty and disorganisation. Simultaneously, it had to meet, with access to medical care no longer dependent on the means of the patient, an immense pent-up demand for treatment. This backlog of needs, accumulated during the war and its uneasy aftermath, was most vividly depicted by the demand for spectacle, dentures, hearing aids and other postponable adjuncts to better health (Abel-Smith and Titmuss, 1956). To those with little sense of history it was this that gave the NHS a bad name.

Against this background, it would indeed have been surprising if the NHS had not been able to show marked improvements in many spheres of activity. Certainly, in quantitative terms, the baseline from which it started was a low one. There was so much waiting to be done and, with the removal of the financial barrier to medical care in 1948, needs and the expectation of the standard at which they might now be met, hitherto submerged or inarticulate, came to the surface. And so were crystallised many of the deeper problems concerning the role of medicine and the profession in modern society. All this has to be remembered, if complacency is to be avoided, in interpreting the verdict of the Guillebaud Report on the performance of the NHS during its first seven years.

Nor, if we push the analysis further back in time, is it easy to make comparisons with the standard of medical care in the 1930s. Critics of the NHS have rarely made explicit the criteria of value they have in mind in drawing comparisons over time. In failing to do so they have, of course, avoided the question as to whether it is possible to make comparisons in many important respects with conditions in the 1930s. There are now more variables in the equation of medical care; science has penetrated the art of medicine at so many points and changed the relativities of skill, knowledge and practice. As functions have changed, so have the relativities of status and reward within the profession itself.

* * * * *

Has the standard or quality of medical care provided by the general practitioner under the NHS deteriorated, compared with that provided during the 1930s under the mixed system of private practice and National Health Insurance panel practice for insured workers? Have general practitioners had to deal with a great increase in demand from patients? Is it true that they no longer function as family doctors, whereas in the 1930s they did? These are typical of the questions which are invariably raised whenever the effects of the NHS on general practice are discussed. The main emphasis thus falls on the general practitioners. They are the pivots of attraction in all the controversy that has surrounded the NHS since its inception. Their future role in the changing field of medical care is the most difficult one to discern. While science has strengthened the prestige and position of the hospital and given it an assured place in the community, it has simultaneously disturbed and, to some extent, made uncertain the role of the general practitioner. Yet, in Britain at least, general practitioners still remain in the frontline in meeting the need for medical care.

I believe that the NHS has made a beginning in the process of establishing a social framework in which the great majority of general practitioners, gradually assimilating the benefits of scientific medicine, may find a more assured and satisfying role than was their lot before

1948. It is, fundamentally, a problem of adjusting to the challenge of scientific medicine; to the changing balance of physical and mental ill-health; to the rising standard of expectations of medical care from a more articulate, health-conscious society. As many are coming to recognise, these adjustments involve the reform of medical education.

* * * * *

Ever since 1948, there has been much dispute about the adequacy of rewards for doctors taking part in the NHS (*British Medical Journal*, 1957, ii, supplement 54). To a substantial extent, this has been a dispute about differentials: the constant attempts of the consultants to keep well ahead of the general practitioners and the equally constant attempts of general practitioners to narrow the differences. On what basis should society fix these rewards, once they are no longer mainly settled by the play of the market, and how should they be distributed among the different branches of the profession and in relation to services rendered? One thing at least can be said with a fair degree of assurance. The introduction of the NHS meant the adoption by the government of a policy of 'levelling-up' for general practitioners. There had been, according to the Spens Committee (1946), which surveyed the earnings of doctors in 1936-38, too many general practitioners with low incomes. This proportion, for those at the ages of peak earning capacity (40 to 45), was put at 40%. An analysis of the figures suggests that private practice was much less remunerative in the 1930s than most people were aware of then or imagine today. Not only were 'bad debts' probably substantial during the years of heavy unemployment, but many people were no doubt reluctant to see a doctor, either because they could not pay or because they already owed the doctor money. Only the existence of National Health Insurance capitation fees saved many general practitioners in industrial areas from poverty. Thus, the Spens Committee "had no doubt that low incomes have, in fact, been a source of grave worry to many general practitioners and must have prejudiced their efficiency".

Despite the official attacks on the NHS by the representatives of the profession, it has in practice turned out to be a most attractive proposition among those desirous of allowing a professional career. Since 1948, all the medical schools in Britain have been flooded with applications. Using the old-fashioned criteria of supply and demand, it would not seem that the profession as a whole is dissatisfied with the prospects and rewards offered to medical men and women under the NHS.

Whatever else may be said about the NHS, it can at least be concluded that, under the new regime, doctors have prospered. But this prosperity has brought with it some social problems: problems of determining the size of the medical profession in the future; of how to select those to be trained as doctors; and of settling their future rewards from public funds. These questions, which cannot be left to the profession alone to solve, were obliquely referred to in picturesque language by R.J.V. Pulvertaft, Professor of Clinical Pathology in the University of London.

> It is not surprising that the opportunity of belonging without expense to the most lucrative profession outside the black market has attracted a flood of applications, far exceeding the vacancies in schools or the requirements of medicine.... This thirst to succour suffering humanity must make all but the cynic blush with pride; but even the most unsuspicious mind must wonder whether a method of medical recruitment which involves no personal sacrifice, still less hardship, for anyone attracts the right men and women.... It is well to remember that the dispensation of national patronage is vested in remarkably few hands. All these candidates come forward with very similar educational qualifications and the eulogies of pedagogues; a handful of deans, with or often without committees, bestows largesse and selects the doctors of tomorrow (Pulvertaft, 1952, vol ii, p 839).

* * * * *

Financial security is not, however, the only attraction to those who now engage in or hope to enter general practice. To most doctors, it is probably of less importance than the conditions under which they work and the kind of relationships they have with their patients and their colleagues.

Fundamental to them all is the question of clinical freedom: the right, as a trusted professional servant, to treat one's patient to the best of one's ability without interference or dictation, and subject only to the ethical code of behaviour laid down by the profession as a whole. There is no doubt that many doctors in Britain saw, in the coming of the NHS, a threat to clinical freedom. The state, through its influence over the earnings and financial status of doctors, could reduce them to poverty and thus make them subservient to the will of the politician or administrator. This fear has not materialised.

Another fear among general practitioners was that their security as doctors might be jeopardised if their services were dispensed with for some reason or other by the Ministry of Health. Safeguards were written into the Health Service Act and an independent National Health Service Tribunal was set up with a legal chairman appointed by the Lord Chancellor. This tribunal is concerned with complaints made by patients against practitioners and thus plays an important role in matters of discipline. It has the power to retain, reinstate and remove the name of a doctor from the list of NHS practitioners or to exact some lesser penalty, such as a fine. Although it is not concerned with the redress of patients' grievances, the real issues with which it has to deal are clearly related to the efficiency of the NHS.

The working of this tribunal has been considered, along with many others, by the Committee on Administrative Tribunals and Enquiries. Their report, while emphasising the need for the utmost care in any matters which affect professional reputations, did, however, make a number of recommendations. The Committee thought that, in general, the tribunal should sit in public; that the right of appeal to the Minister should be abolished, and that at some stages in the procedure, complainants should be given official assistance in presenting their cases.

The editor of the *Lancet*, T.F. Fox, concisely summed up the lessons of this experience in lecturing on 'professional freedom' when he said: "I would say, that, in joining the public service, doctors have been given as much security of tenure as is justified in the public interests. They run very little risk of losing their contracts through arbitrary action by the Minister or his servants; their fears of being directed to practise in under-doctored areas have not been realised; and there is still free choice of doctor by patient and of patient by doctor. Another important safeguard of their professional freedom is the declaration that they may speak and write as they think fit" (Fox, 1951, p 173).

Finally, on this question of professional freedom, there was the fear of administrative control or interference in the treatment of patients and other clinical matters. At the annual meeting of the British Medical Association in 1955, Talbot Rogers, an influential general practitioner, said: "Speaking for the general practitioners ... after seven years' experience of the new service ... they had achieved a remarkable degree of clinical and administrative freedom" (*British Medical Journal*, 1955, supplement ii, p 119). Nor has this freedom, apparently greater than under the old National Insurance system, been purchased at the price of less satisfactory relationships with patients.

* * * * *

No discussion of professional freedom in the field of medicine can be concluded without mention of doctors' freedom to serve their patients according to their medical needs. The Act of 1946 greatly enlarged this freedom – particularly in respect of the treatment of women and children, older people, disabled people and chronically ill people, and the middle-income groups in the community. No longer did the doctors have to ask themselves whether the patient could afford this or that treatment; whether they should ask the patient to come again; what the patient would think of them as people and as doctors if they did so; whether the patient could afford this drug or that special service; how long they could wait before making a definitive diagnosis; and whether it would be cheaper for the patient to go to hospital or be treated at home; and whether or not it was of financial consequence to the doctor and to the patient to call in a consultant, to seek evidence from X-ray and laboratory tests, to advise surgery, or to allow the 'wisdom of the body' to reassert itself.

This enlargement of freedom for the British doctor to treat patients according to their medical needs came at a critical period in the history of medicine. By 1948, the tide of scientific and technological change was in full flood. One of the consequences of change was to push up pharmaceutical and other costs at a rapid rate. Another was to change the relativities of skill and function as between the general practitioner, the consultant and the hospital. A third was to make the older general practitioners feel more insecure and uncertain about the performance of their functions, and thus to fear the coming of the NHS with more anxiety than perhaps they would have done if scientific change had not been so strong and pervasive at that time.

Within the last 10 to 15 years [up to 1958], the potential sphere of work of general practitioners has been extended. They can now treat diseases which for a time they had lost to the hospital: principally pneumonia, pernicious anaemia, most subcutaneous purulent infections, and most infections of the ears, pharynx, lungs and bowels (*Lancet*, 1954, vol I, p 659). "Today the practitioner in the gloomiest slum practice can treat pneumonia more effectively than the most eminent specialist was able to do before the war" (Taylor, 1954, p 551).

The total effect of all these changes has made it possible for general practitioners to do more or to do less for their patients; to be personally responsible for more or less serious illness among their patients; to do more or less preventive work; in short, to be relatively better or relatively worse doctors (Hadfield, 1953). We see, in this way, how science, by enlarging the potential field of choice and action, simultaneously enlarges the potential for individual freedom. The NHS in Britain could not ensure that doctors, now invested with these greater powers and potentialities, would choose overnight to be 'better' doctors; all it could do was to provide that particular framework of social resources within which potentially 'better' medicine might be more easily chosen and practised.

* * * * *

It should be emphasised that remarkably little is known about the institution of private medical care before 1948. For the first decade of the 20th century, there is some information. We know that, before the introduction of Lloyd George's Health Insurance Act in 1911, the standard of medical care for the vast majority of the population was abysmally low by present-day standards. Competitive under-cutting, fee-splitting, canvassing for patients and other unethical practices were widespread. Most doctors were extremely poorly paid and worked under degrading conditions. The out-patient departments of voluntary hospitals, described by the Webbs (1910, p 134) as "mammoth shops, run by underpaid doctors, for the mass treatment of symptoms with free bottles of medicine" (chiefly *saccharuum ustum* or brown sugar and water) were regarded by general practitioners as unfair competitors, threatening their main source of income (Hardy, 1901, pp 20-1, 49-55). For the years between 1911 and 1948, we know very little about what doctors were paid by private patients, what unpaid bills there were, what services were given, how much work doctors had to do, what the pattern of prescribing was, and so forth.

The NHS has not had the effect of taking away the right of the general practitioner to function as a 'family doctor'. In the past, 'family doctoring' only existed for a small section of the population, chiefly the inhabitants of relatively isolated rural areas and middle- and upper-middle-class patients. After 1948, with the removal of the financial barriers, it became more possible for general practitioners to function as family doctors. Some of the changing of doctors that appears to have gone on in the early years of the NHS may simply have reflected the desire of families to get all their members on to the list of one doctor. Unfortunately, and in the absence of any research into the reality of 'family doctoring', this movement seems to have been interpreted by the British Medical Association as 'abuse' (in the sense of competitively playing off one doctor against another). Pressure was, therefore, brought to bear on the Ministry of Health to make it less easy for patients to change their doctors.

It has been widely believed, especially among the profession, that the introduction of the NHS led to a large increase in the average number of items of service required from general practitioners by each patient per year. A detailed examination of all the published reports on the subject – including five large statistical studies on National Health Insurance before 1939 and six or so NHS studies after 1948 of varying quality – do not confirm this belief. The most trustworthy data for the latter period show, for 1949-50, a total general practitioner consultation rate for both sexes at all ages over 16 of 4.62 (attendances 3.00; visits 1.62). For men only aged 16 to 64 (probably a better index to use for comparison with pre-war data), the rate was 3.60 (attendances 2.77; visits 0.83). Two extensive studies of National Health Insurance demand in the 1930s, carried out on behalf of the British Medical Association, give rates of 5.02 and 5.10 (attendances, roughly 3.80; visits, roughly 1.25). The only conclusion that can be drawn from these and other statistical materials is that, on average and contrary to public belief, demand has not increased under the NHS and may indeed have fallen. Although comparisons with American experience are almost impossible, there is a little evidence that demand may be higher in the US and that it has been rising.

What we do not know from these British studies is the level of demand from the private sector in the 1930s. There is some evidence to suggest that demand from middle-class and professional groups increased after 1948.

It is also relevant to bring into account other evidence which shows the following when comparing the present situation with that in the 1930s:

(a) a decline in the average number of persons per general practitioner in a substantial number of areas;
(b) an improvement in the geographical distribution of doctors in relation to needs;
(c) a decline in the amount of night-visiting by general practitioners;
(d) a remarkable growth in the adoption of voluntary rota systems for evening, weekend and other duty periods; and
(e) a decrease in the number of statutory certificates issued per 100 patients per year.

Finally, I come to the question of quality of care by general practitioners. It is by far the most difficult question, not only because of the theoretical problem of defining what one means by 'quality', but also on account of assessing it in practice. While it is one thing for a medical observer to identify really bad general practitioner work among selected individual doctors at a given point in time, it is quite another thing to make comparisons over time between random groups of doctors. No scientific observations were made on these matters in the 1930s. There is some documentary evidence to suggest that for many people receiving treatment under National Health Insurance, Public Assistance and Workmen's Compensation practice, the quality of care, by the standards we expect in the 1950s, was very low (Levy, 1944). Hardly anything is known about private practice except the evidence of such indirect indices as high rates of tonsillectomy, inadequate prenatal care, excessive surgical interference in childbearing, and too frequent use of operative procedures in small, general practitioner hospitals. In short, when it is alleged that the quality of care by general practitioners has deteriorated under the NHS, there is little to support such statements, except impressions and memories of past experience.

What evidence there is could in theory point the other way. The supreme requisite of good practitioner care is time and many general practitioners have, on average, more time to spend with each patient than they had before 1948, if they wish to use it that way, and more time for diagnosis, the foundation of all good medical care. Against this consideration has to be set the unknown effects of six other critically important variables:

(a) the educational equipment and clinical skill of the doctor,
(b) the capacity to understand sick people;
(c) the range, content and power of the scientific aids available to the general practitioner;
(d) the nature and extent of contacts with professional colleagues;
(e) the facilities available for dealing with the social aspects of ill-health; and
(f) the incidence of ill-health, mental and physical, and the norms of expectation or awareness of what constitutes 'good medical care' among the population as a whole (Morris, 1957).

The role that these and other variables play in the total equation has changed. Time still remains, however, as a factor of supreme importance. Science and the recognition of the mental component in ill-health may perhaps have heightened its value to doctor and patient alike. Nor is this truth in any way dimmed by the fact that the general practitioner today is responsible, as some recent studies have shown, for the treatment of a substantial amount of serious organic and infectious disease.

We must, therefore, look for some more searching tool than generalities about 'abuse' and 'deteriorating standards'. If the NHS did not exist in Britain today, would there be more or less misuse of the antibiotics, the barbiturates and other chemical tranquillisers; more or less unnecessary surgery; earlier or later access to medical care; more or fewer hasty, untested diagnoses; more or fewer unethical practices; and more or fewer income, class, age, sex and geographical differentials in respect of all these and other factors? I suggest that these are the kind of questions which are more likely to stimulate a search for reliable evidence.

The ethics and economics of medical care

The notion that medical care requires to be deliberately organised through the medium of a third party is not a new one in the history of medicine. In the days of Hippocrates, salaried physicians were appointed by the community to treat the sick without a fee. The Romans employed many of their physicians and surgeons on the same basis. Nor was it unknown among third parties for the method to be used of paying doctors on a capitation basis. The introduction by the British of a free-on-demand health service in 1948 was not, therefore, in its essential principles a novel event.

Yet it is now being regarded by a growing number of economists, supported in London by the Institute of Economic Affairs and in the US by the American Medical Association, as a unique aberration. This is attributed to what one economist, D.S. Lees (1961), describes as "a strange neglect of general economic principles". In his pamphlet, *Health through choice*, he attempts to repair this omission. Applying classical economic theory to the NHS and its development since 1948, he postulates an alternative to organised medical care – namely, the invisible hand of the private market. The fundamental choice, he argues, lies between individual consumer sovereignty and collective arrangements. The function of consumers is to choose, bargain and buy – not to organise supply. No third party is presumed to intervene or is required to intervene in the private transactions between two people – patient and doctor.

One of the assumptions implicit in Lees' thesis is that economic principles were not neglected in the past in the relations between doctor and patient in Britain. This suggests, therefore, the existence at some time of a state of affairs in which the consumer was sovereign and no third parties intervened in the financial dialogue between buyer and seller. How much historical truth there is in this proposition depends, of course, on the period selected for comparative purposes. Something akin to the model of a free market may have prevailed in the centuries of folk-medicine just as it still does today among certain peoples in Africa and Asia. We know from the studies of social anthropologists that one of the essential characteristics of folk or non-rational medicine is that of shared knowledge between patient and doctor. It therefore fulfils one of the requisites of a free market: the buyer should not be placed in a subordinate position to the seller.

Dialogue and transaction take place – or can presumably take place – on the basis of some equality of knowledge. But if, as was often the case, the purveyor of medical care also had priestly functions, the analogy with the market broke down, as it may do today when the doctor assumes an apostolic role. The consumer thus relinquishes the claim to sovereignty. Submission to higher authority demands behaviour which is inappropriate and ineffective in the market place.

Such comparisons with the distant past or with certain cultures are therefore not particularly helpful in the testing of economic theory. Perhaps the most appropriate period to select for the examination of Lees' assumption is that immediately preceding 1911 and the advent of organised National Health Insurance. Even here, however, the model of consumer sovereignty does not fit at all easily for the mass of patients and general practitioners.

Apart from the employment of many practitioners under the Poor Law during the early years of the 20th century, there were also large numbers engaged in club and contract practice. Free choice of doctor did not obtain in these conditions, and the doctors were paid by third parties either on a salaried basis or by piece-rates. Professionally, their work was often strictly controlled by the administrators and lay committees of voluntary associations, insurance companies and Poor Law authorities. It is probable that there were proportionately more salaried general practitioners during this period of presumed free market conditions in medical care than there are today under the NHS. "The cause of these evils is the advantage which non-medical organizations are able to take of the competition between individual medical parishioners" (British Medical Association, 1905, p 28). This helps to explain what Eckstein (1955) has noted, that the Association was then far more hostile to private than to public control. Hence its objection in these circumstances to payment by piece-rates. Some 50 years later, much the same conclusion was reached by the President of the American Hospital Association who remarked in 1959 that public control over voluntary hospitals was to be preferred to private control (Somers and Somers, 1961).

Only among a section of the profession do we find from the historical studies that have been made anything resembling free-market conditions prevailing during the Edwardian period (Abel-Smith, 1964). Competition for patients, an essential attribute of a free market, was inevitably accompanied as theory would imply by widespread fee-splitting, commission-taking, canvassing, the dispensation of 'secret remedies', and the employment of unqualified assistants. Monopolistic conditions did not then obtain for there was much competition from the medically unqualified and various other purveyors of 'secret remedies'. Outside the Poor Law and club and contract practice, the price of medical care was not administered or regulated in the sense understood by modern students of imperfect competition.

It would seem, therefore, that Lees' assumption of free market conditions operating without the intervention of third parties has only limited validity in respect of the period before organised health insurance in 1911. In so far as the thesis does hold, however, we should note the implications of consumer sovereignty for professional standards of medical behaviour and medical ethics. These are matters which Lees does not discuss, nor are they referred to in another economic analysis by Jewkes and Jewkes (1961, p 36): "It is reasonable to suppose that even without a National Health Service, Britain would have enjoyed after 1948 medical services more ample and better distributed than those which existed before the war". No doubt their reason for omitting any consideration of professional ethics is to be found in the statement by another economist, F.G. Dickinson, Head of the American Medical Association's Bureau of Medical Economic Research in 1956: "The doctor is essentially a small businessman. He is selling his services so is as much in business as anyone else who sells a commodity" (Carter, 1958, p 88).

It would thus follow that, if a private medical market place, envisaged by these Conservative and Liberal economists, is to operate effectively in Britain, it should be peopled by the kind of doctors described by D. Lowell Kelly of the University of Michigan (1957, pp 195-6). Reporting on the personality characteristics of medical students, he said that they revealed "remarkably little interest in the welfare of human beings . . . the *typical* [author's italics] young physician ... is generally not inclined to participate in community activities unless these contribute to his income ... he is still essentially an entrepreneur".

The logic of the case presented by Lees and Jewkes would thus appear to demand quite different considerations in the selection and training of medical students in Britain than those which are accepted today. Such students would need to be taught to give preferential treatment to consumers who will pay most for what they have to sell; consumers who are presumed, as a result of the free play of the market, to be more worthwhile in genetic or productive terms. This proposition is akin to the thesis advance by Ffrangcon Roberts in *The cost of health* (1952), a "brilliantly argued" book according to Lees.

In embracing the market system, doctors would thus relinquish their role as "centres of moral life" (Durkheim, 1957, p 26). Logically again, it would thus follow that society could no longer depend on doctors to give truthful information about their patients, or even information as reliable as one normally expects from the average shopkeeper.

* * * * *

What makes even more speculative these attempts to apply classical economic theory to systems of medical care is the advent of science. In terms of diagnosis and therapy, the scientific revolution gathered momentum after the discovery of prontosil in 1935. The tremendous impact on medical practice and professional ethics of scientific and technological developments during the past two decades [1940s and 1950s] has been described by many writers. Its effects on the doctor–patient relationship may be summarised under four related heads:

(i)   a great increase in specialisation and in the division of medical labour;
(ii)   the proliferation at an accelerating pace of more and more technical and paramedical instruments of diagnosis and therapy;
(iii) an apparent rise in the price of medical care continually exceeding the rise in the price of other consumer goods and services; and
(iv)   in consequence of these and other trends, an immense enlargement, in relative terms, in the average patient's ignorance about medical matters.

The more it becomes a science like thermodynamics and nuclear physics, the more will medicine place patients in a position of inequality not unlike that they occupied before the Renaissance.

Yet Lees argues, in drawing an analogy between the role of the doctor and the functioning of washing machines, that, in both cases, the consumer has to call in the expert. In concluding, therefore, that medical care is no different from such commodities, he fails to make three distinctions: first, between services and objects; second, between events that are a threat to life and those that are not; and third, between costs that can be estimated in advance and predicted over time, and costs that cannot be so estimated and predicted. To disregard these distinctions means, in technical terms, therefore, that ordinal analysis applied to consumer demand equates mink coats with Caesarean operations in childbirth. At given rates, they are assumed to be interchangeable.

It may be objected, of course, that there are many other parallels for calling in (or relying on) the expert. Engine drivers and garage mechanics who do not do their jobs properly are a threat to life, but trains and cars are different from human minds and bodies. This is a value judgment, but it is one which few would dispute. We can decide to stop running a car, but most of us cannot decide to stop breathing. Nor do cars have babies or have to care for other cars. Nor do we, as ignorant lay people, always know that we want medical care until we have 'consumed' it.

All these imponderable and quantitatively immeasurable factors have to be taken into account in any attempt to equate medical care with mink coats or car repairs.

We can also examine these matters, not only by making comparisons in historical terms but also by looking at contemporary experiences in other countries. The obvious one to select for this purpose is the US, the citadel of 'free enterprise medicine'.

The notions of consumer sovereignty, individual freedom of choice, variety versus conformity, and centralised control versus the free market, have been increasingly applied in recent years to other social services such as education and housing, and social security as well as medical care. The case for the market has been ably presented by economists and other writers on behalf of the Conservative and Liberal parties.

These services, collectively organised by the state, are seen as a temporary economic phenomenon peculiar to a specific historical phase in the development of large-scale industrial societies. They were needed as social supports when the masses were poor; in times of war; and when the future of capitalism was uncertain. These conditions, it is argued, no longer obtain. Thus the 'welfare state', after another celebrated example, should wither away, and more and more people should have resort to a self-regulating market – to quote Lees, "the superior means of registering preferences". It is more sensitive than government; it automatically corrects for mistakes in supply; it enables individuals to adjust their consumption and saving more easily; it provides more variety and thus increases consumer satisfactions; it is less bureaucratic and, administratively, more efficient. Private responsibility should thus replace public paternalism. These are the main arguments and appealing phrases for removing the present state impediments to a free market in education, housing, social security and medical care. Is this thesis supported by the behaviour of the medical care market in the US?

* * * * *

We must begin with the American consumers. From their point of view, one of the more obvious and striking facts of life is the continuing rise in the cost of medical care. Since 1948, it has risen much more than in Britain. The rise began in the early 1940s and has steadily accelerated. Between 1947 and the end of the 1950s, the cost of medical care services rose more than twice as fast as all items in the Bureau of Labor Statistics Consumer Price Index. By June 1960, it was rising three times as fast. By far the steepest rise has been registered by the price of hospital rooms and group hospital insurance premiums. These are now rising at the rate of over 7% per year, or twice as fast as the national income. All the evidence points to continuing price inflation, particularly because of the growing shortage of doctors and nurses, the advent of more profit-making hospitals as a source of capital gains, the trend from domicilary to hospital care, and other factors.

The price indices do not show changes in the quantity or quality of medical care purchased. In 15 years, total expenditure on health and medical care has steadily risen and now [1963] stands at something over 5% of the gross national product (GNP). Included in this total, personal consumption on private medical care rose from 2.9% of GNP in 1947 to 3.7% in 1958. These figures show that effective demand has been increasing, but it is hard to say what proportions of the additional expenditures are due to: the increasing population – particularly among older people; price inflation; higher administrative and selling costs; more items of service per head; better quality services; and duplicated and underutilised services, and other factors.

The problem of disentangling the respective contributions of all these factors is one of great complexity. It is much too simple to suggest that, if the Americans are spending a higher proportion of their GNP on medical care, it necessarily confirms the private market as superior in supplying a better service in quality as well as quantity. The reverse might be true, if many Americans are today being forced to pay more for the same measured service. As one example, in 1959, some $750 million was spent on drug promotion or nearly one quarter of personal consumption spending on drug preparations and sundries. This proportion was considerably higher than 10 years earlier.

No one who devotes any serious attention to the vast literature on medical care in the US in recent years can fail to observe the many signs and symptoms of frustration and consumer dissatisfaction. According to a report to Congress (Roberts, 1959), "the supply of available medical care, in terms of medical personnel and medical facilities, is declining in relation to population growth and rising health consciousness. Shortages of supply exist already and will grow more serious in the future....".

The number of hospital beds per 1,000 population dropped from 9.7 in 1948 to 9.2 in 1962 (Brewster and Seldowitz, 1962). In England and Wales over the same period, the number of staffed beds rose from 10.2 to 10.3. Moreover, the American figures include a spectacular growth in the number of proprietary and profit-making hospitals in various areas – most of them small and inadequately staffed and equipped – despite the technical rationale for large units (Gramm, 1962). Investment in these hospitals is said to be "particularly attractive for investors seeking capital gains" (Hamilton, 1961, p 95).

One developer, writing in the *Wall Street Journal*, envisages a coast-to-coast chain of such hospitals, viewing them as a "bread and butter item – just like food stores" (Seymour, 1959, p 1). Some of these hospitals are connected with pharmacies, and in 1961, it was reported that at least 450 doctors were whole or part owners of pharmacies in the state of California alone (*Los Angeles Times*, 21 May 1961).

In February 1962, the US Public Health Service, Preliminary Report, reported that the country faced a shortage of more than one million "acceptable" hospital beds. There is serious over-building of hospitals and gross duplication of expensive equipment in some areas, growing shortages in others, and a general trend towards greater maldistribution in important sectors of medical care. One part of the price of non-planning – a 26% average non-occupancy rate in short-term general hospital beds in 1957 – cost American consumers $3.5 billion in idle investment and $625 million in operating costs (Brown, 1959).

At the same time, the shortage of less expensive long-term facilities – for example, mental hospital beds – grew worse throughout the 1950s. There is no evidence that this problem of maldistribution is being automatically corrected by 'natural' market forces. One study (Roberts, 1962) in Michigan has indicated that $5 million a year is wasted in that state because of 'uneconomical hospitalisation' and lack of coordinated action. While 'unnatural' or governmental forces have undoubtedly brought about an improvement in the geographical distribution of doctors and medical resources in Britain since 1948, there has been little change over the same period in the striking disparities in the state ratios of physicians to population in America (Somers, 1961).

Other signs of consumer dissatisfaction and of the failure of corrective market forces are to be found in the growth of various forms of medico-scientific charlatanism, resort to the corner drugstore, chiropractors, naturopaths, and the steeply rising costs of malpractice insurance. In California, the young doctor has now [1963] to pay around $820 a year for such insurance; one practising doctor in four has been the target of a malpractice suit or claim. In Britain, the comparable figure is about $6. Malpractice suits are thought to be a symptom of a breakdown in doctor–patient relationships.

A nationwide study commissioned by the American Medical Association in 1958 reported that 44% of all the people interviewed had had 'unfavourable experiences' with doctors, 32% of them so unsatisfactory that they said they would not return to the same doctor (Somers, 1961).

* * * * *

The general conclusion that many students of medical care are now formulating is that the forces normally presumed in America to produce acceptable allocations of resources are singularly inoperative in the case of hospital services. Profit maximisation is clearly not the force directing the behaviour of general hospitals organised as independent units under the control of self-perpetuating boards of directors. Nor is it the force which is making hospital care more and more expensive for many people. American experience does not, therefore, support Lees' advocacy of transferring hospitals to private ownership on the grounds that such ownership would keep down costs, expose poor performance, redress imbalances and be more sensitive to consumer demands.

Economists in Britain have yet to learn that, on both the demand and supply side, the market for hospital services is, to say the least, unusual. Theoretical assumptions about demand have to be revised because of the almost complete consumer ignorance both of the need for and the quality of hospital care – particularly surgical treatment. Price competition in these circumstances does not exist. Patients are told to go to hospital and, in the US, to that institution at which their physician has staff privileges. Moreover, the rapid disappearance of the general practitioner means that more and more people may be losing an essential patient liberty – the advice, protection and defence which the general practitioners are in a position to give their patients. This role of standing between the patient, the hospital and over-specialisation increases in importance as scientific medicine becomes more complex, more functionally divided and potentially more lethal. These developments are enlarging the need for the detached, non-specialist diagnostician – the doctor who can interpret scientific medicine and the processes of diagnosis and treatment to the patient according to the circumstances of each case, and without any functional or financial commitment to a specialised area of practice.

In the absence of this relationship with a personal, generalised doctor, the patient in the US has increasingly to resort to self-diagnosis. "It is generally recognised that America is the most over-medicated, most over-operated, and most over-inoculated country in the world" (Ratner, 1962). The patient has to decide, when to 'feel ill', which – if any – specialist to consult. Is the patient – or can the patient be – equipped with the requisite knowledge? Should specialists be expected to perform this generalised role and are they, in their turn, better equipped to do so than the general practitioner?

In the American situation, the specialist may be the answer in certain individual circumstances, but these can rarely be known or predicted in advance by the consumer. If, moreover, there is a danger of the general practitioner masquerading, so to speak, as a specialist (as there undoubtedly is in the US) the patient will understandably seek the 'genuine' specialist and thereby be driven to self-diagnosis. Many other forces – cultural, economic and quasi-professional – also add to the attractions of the scientific 'miracle', specialism and the wonders of hospital medicine.

What we have to ask, therefore, is whether this system of medical care, beginning with patient self-diagnosis, is likely to result in better (more effective) quality of care. In considering this question, we must not forget the importance of both time and opportunity costs. Any definition of quality must take account of (i) the time that elapses between the onset of symptoms and complete recovery, and (ii) benefits forgone by the patient during this period of illness. Lees, in maintaining that there are "no differences in principle between medical care and other goods" (1961, p 24), overlooks these factors and, consequently, leaves it to be assumed that, in conditions of free-enterprise medicine, the processes of self-diagnosis and self-selection of the right specialist can be equated with the market choice between cabbages and cauliflowers. Moreover, if consumers are ignorant or restrictive practices also lead to 'market imperfections', according to Lees, these should be got rid of by government.

This can only mean that consumers of medical care must have as much knowledge of specialist medicine as consumers of cabbages have about vegetables. Lees does not face the problem of educating consumers in medical science – let alone the annual cost of malpractice claims estimated in the US at $45 million to $50 million (Somers, 1961) – nor the implications of breaking restrictive practices among an occupational group which must then, according to the logic of the market, lose its claim to be a self-controlling profession.

Another imperfection – limitation of free choice – which most observers of trends in American medical care have noted results from the pressures which are increasingly forcing resort to hospital medicine. One comes from the trend towards specialisation and the fragmentation of medical practice; there are now in the US about 50 types of physician. If this trend continues at its present pace, the overwhelming majority of physicians will be specialists in 20 years (US Public Health Service, September 1961). Another force is expressed by the decline in home care and home visits. Only about 8% of all physician–patient consultations now take place in the home. On the analogy of the market, the sick have to go to an office – or a series of offices some of which are in hospitals – or to an outpatient clinic. Is this a choice that consumers have voluntarily made?

In England and Wales, despite a relatively smaller rural population, over one third of all such consultations under the NHS take place in the patient's home.

Private hospital insurance is perhaps the most powerful force leading to increased hospitalisation. The availability of partial prepayment of hospital bills and the absence of cover for all medical bills has resulted, according to many surveys, in unnecessary hospital stays, unnecessary diagnostic procedures, unnecessary treatments and surgical operations (Hayes, 1954). One nationwide survey in 1952-53 reported that 22% of the operations were performed by doctors without any surgical specialisation and another 27% by doctors who were neither board-certified nor Fellows of the American College of Surgeons (Somers, 1961). Another study from Columbia University in 1962 showed that over one third of all hysterectomies performed were unnecessary (M. Kaplan, quoting from R.E. Trussell, *New York Times*, 11 May 1962).

The imbalances and distortions created by private hospital insurance systems often contradict the principles of good medical care and consumer choice. They must inevitably flourish in market situations in which science has increased the relative ignorance and sense of helplessness among consumers. There is a "great financial premium on organic diagnosis" because most so-called insurance contracts do not pay for mental illness. The doctor with a patient whose illness is basically mental must choose between "making a complete diagnosis, as a result of which his patient will suffer financially, or making an incomplete diagnosis so that his patient may derive greater benefits" (Poinstard, 1958, p 42). Lees is in favour of this dichotomy. He maintains that mental health should be the responsibility of the state. He does not, however, explain why modern medical care for psychological illness is less susceptible to the superior forces of the market than medical care for physical illness – if they can, in the light of advancing knowledge, be operationally separated.

Their inability to make choices leads some consumers to demand 'their rights' written in partial prepayment contracts: X number of days in hospital, access to an expensive drug, three X-rays a year, and so on. Similarly, some doctors put up their charges when they learn that consumers have already 'bought' particular units of service. A rise in the price of an appendectomy – which has been 'bought' but which may or may not be necessary – will cost the consumer nothing in the short run or until the policy comes round for renewal (Taylor, 1956). Other 'commercial' costs, which the consumer cannot control, reside in the widespread practices between doctors of fee-splitting, rebates, payoffs, commissions and ghost surgery (Hawley, 1952).

In an era when science is demanding more medical teamwork, the problem grows of how to divide responsibility for the patient and how to divide fees from the patient and or their third party agent.

* * * * *

The cumulative result of these and other unneutral forces in the American medical marketplace in shifting the emphasis away from preventive and community medicine is leading to a cost crisis in the hospitals and in private health insurance. Somers and Somers, in their authoritative study (1961, p 407), came to the conclusion that this problem "appears to have reached the point where it threatens the possibility of further progress…. Consumer resentment could menace the survival of private health insurance". The free market, which Lees tells us exists in the US, has failed to call forth an increase in supply to lower consumer costs.

Yet, in attempting to cut costs, the system has gone almost as far as it can in rejecting, cancelling and cutting off the bad risks and their families – the old, the mentally ill, the chronically ill, the unemployed and redundant, the disabled, widows and many other vulnerable groups.

The premium structure of voluntary carriers is being 'commercialised' while the insurance companies (who are increasingly leading the field) have demonstrated their inability to cover the aged and other bad risks. The administrative and commission costs of insurance companies for individual policies rose from 42% in 1948 to 52% in 1958 (Somers, 1961). Consumers now get less than half their dollars back in medical care.

The medical cost problems of a substantial section of the American population cannot now be solved by insurance carriers; the victory of experience-rating over community-rating has been too overwhelming. As MacLean, former president of the Blue Cross Association, said:

> A lifetime's experience has led me at last to conclude that the costs of care of the aged cannot be met, unaided, by the mechanisms of insurance or prepayment as they exist today. The aged simply cannot afford to buy from any of these the scope of care that is required, nor do the stern competitive realities permit any carrier, whether non-profit or commercial, to provide benefits which are adequate at a price which is feasible for any but a small proportion of the aged. (MacLean, 1960, p 2)

When we turn to consider the supply of doctors, all the signs point to the failure of the market. Yet Lees argued – without recourse to any comparative facts – that the market would work very differently from government. It would produce more doctors: the "whole process would be anonymous, continuous and pervasive" (Lees, 1961, p 46). Between 1949 and 1960, the ratio of all types of practising doctors in Britain per head of the population rose by 21%. In the US, it fell by 2%.

American medical education has not had to face such a serious situation since the Flexner Report in 1910. The quantity and quality of applicants to medical schools has been steadily declining and many schools are having great difficulty in filling their first-year places with well-qualified students. The 1959 Report of the Surgeon General's Consultant Group on Medical Education shows that the US will be confronted with a grave shortage of doctors in the decade ahead (US Public Health Service, October 1959). A shortage has been predicted for many years. The 'delicate mechanism' of market forces shows no signs of life.

* * * * *

Classical supply and demand analysis may help us to understand the social institutions of very simple medical economies, but it is singularly unhelpful when applied to the immensely complicated play of forces operating in the field of modern scientific medicine. Theoretical short-cuts are no substitute for the slow and painful study of reality. In an age when we are all oppressed with the weight of facts and our own appalling ignorance, such short-cuts appear to offer the prospect

of a grand design and a simple choice of alternative courses of action.
So Lees tells us that the "fundamental issue is whether the supply of
medical care should be based on the principle of consumers'
sovereignty or be made the subject of collective provision".

This is not the issue in the US or in Britain. The American people
are faced – and will continue to be faced in a pluralistic society –
with a complex series of inter-related social, economic and ethical
issues. These issues lie beyond economics and derive ultimately from
one's beliefs of what constitutes the good society. How we organise,
rather than whether we should organise at all, is the question we
should ask of medical care as well as of education, social security and
other social services.

The sociology of health care

Jonathan Barker and Janet Askham

L ike doctors (Charles-Jones et al, 2003), sociologists nowadays tend to specialise in the face of burgeoning knowledge. Dividing their subject according to different criteria, they may develop an almost exclusive focus on, for example, health behaviour, professions, ethnic relations, bureaucracy, institutions or older people. They observe society but are also part of it and even typify it. They have internecine disputes. They apply labels such as 'positivist', 'ethno-methodologist', 'theorist', 'reformist', 'marxist', 'gerontologist' or even 'specialist' to themselves and each other, sometimes in derision or competition. They try to maintain hegemony over their subject and reputation. Except by escaping it to join the ranks of social activists, few manage to liberate themselves from the trammels of their 'profession' and combine due respect for impartial value-free interpretation of data (and academic rigour) with success in reaching out to capture the respect of a wider public (O'Neill, 1972).

* * * * *

For Titmuss, however, this issue did not pose a dilemma. He analysed the world sociologically but did not aspire to be a sociologist, at least not exclusively. He was a common-sense polymath – a general practitioner of social analysis – for whom such boundaries were unnatural constraints on both clear vision and the pursuit of social values. He appeared slight and unassuming, but his lectures set minds alight. They were full of evidence, yet they were overarching. His social data provided him with the spectacles of the generalist observer, rather than the telescope of the specialist. Through them, he reviewed services from the perspective of their social benefit. There were only two limits to his cross–disciplinary exploratory tendency. The first was set by the availability of contemporary knowledge and, especially, firm empirical data, although its very lack spurred him to speculation and foresight. This was a freedom that has eluded many more recent analysts, weighed down with the indigestible mass of data that has emerged, significantly stimulated by him, since his era. In fact, by the time of Titmuss's death in 1973, there was quite a body of 'medical sociological' literature, little of it empirical and most of it American, focusing on doctor–patient relations. This provided grist for a small mill of social scientists proselytising about their discipline (or way of looking at the medical world) in front of neophyte health practitioners. It was part of a process to help to humanise medicine and to enable doctors to understand their patients' health beliefs. Initially attractive for its potential for insights into "patient compliance with medical regimens", the teaching of this early medical sociology grew into a small but significant element in medical education. It also constituted a significant contributor to understanding social factors in ill-health and differential ageing and mortality (see, for example, Coe, 1970; Freeman et al, 1973; and, of more UK relevance, Tuckett, 1976).

The second limit concerned the purpose of social enquiry. For Titmuss, the sole rationale for it was the enhancement of the conditions of people and, especially, the leavening of the inequalities which he observed and which he showed to have dramatic impacts on mortality and morbidity and, thus, the quality and very continuation of life.

It is this commitment to enlightened human welfare that is most highlighted by the four pieces in this part of the book on the sociology of health care. It is a commitment he assumes and expects in his audience. So his analysis of what is wrong with a service, profession or institution starts with a review of how and why it fails to meet such expectations. It is encompassed in his distinction between *welfare state*, which to political economists (and many American ears) implies part of a system of social control, something the state imposes in the context of conflict between the individual, the state and capitalism, and *welfare society*. The latter is more recognisable to observers in the UK who assume its goals are genuinely concerned with the pursuit of humanitarian, even egalitarian, values, and a history built up from Shaftsbury and Booth, through Lloyd George and Beveridge, and which is expressed at its best in Titmuss's altruistic NHS (Titmuss, 1950; Runciman, 1966; Cochrane and Clarke, 1993). For Titmuss, the state was merely the most democratic and trustworthy manager of such a welfare society. It was also the only one that could be trusted to apply generalist principles and to administer in the interests of the whole society. For radical policy analysts today, the focus on inequality is more likely to encompass gender and ethnic differences as well as social class, and with less hope or confidence in the ability of the state to ameliorate them.

The first chapter in this section focuses on the emergence of medicine as science. It records changes that had happened by the end of the first nine years of the NHS, especially the therapeutic revolution which, by then, had added early antibiotics and new immunisations (for example, polio) to public health measures and vaccines of more restricted value (for example, smallpox). These gave family doctors the first real non-surgical weapons (apart from rest, warmth, food, fresh air and the passage of time) against disease. Omitting only a foretaste of the transformation in the understanding of genetics, Titmuss's commentary here is remarkably prescient about the impact of burgeoning medical knowledge on professional specialisation and a doctor's capacity to understand the 'whole patient', especially within his or her whole social context. Here his beam shines on general practice, which had not then emerged into a speciality of family care, of interdisciplinary team leadership or into a pivotal role in selecting (or 'purchasing') specialist diagnostic or treatment options on behalf of (and, ideally, in consultation with) the patient. But this is Titmuss's implied dream, reflecting the belief enshrined in the report on the British Health Services published by Political and Economic Planning in 1937 that the "GP should become recognized as the specialist in diagnosis … [for it is the GP] … alone (who) sees the patient as a person living under certain conditions and not merely as a case" (Herbert, 1939, p 79). In this bridge-building enabling role, transcending disciplinary boundaries, Titmuss was to sociology what his ideal-type GP is to medicine, diagnosing problems for clients and opening bureaucratic doors to better and fairer treatment for them.

Today's much rarer encounters with history's inner-city lock-up GP surgeries – and, in its most extreme example, the horrors of Dr Shipman's murderous capacity to operate unsupervised and unconnected with the mainstream health care system – still remind us of the dangers of failing to build the GP into this pivotal role, based with several colleagues in a well-resourced health centre. This failure deprived the NHS of many years of enhanced primary care and its less fortunate patients of fair access to treatment. Titmuss's description of early deputising services unconnected to records or the personal touch envisaged for the family doctor as, in a positive sense, gate-keeper to decent care, is in marked contrast to recent initiatives in task sharing between professionals. By contrast, there are encouraging recent examples of out-of-hours GP cooperatives (co-ops) and patient access to online and telephone health advice under the auspices of NHS Direct, which complement the role of the family practitioner. Recently, with the recognition and encouragement of private deputising services, the principles underlying the co-ops and the standards expected of them and of GPs themselves have been incorporated into a new GP contract. This has been negotiated to enhance and monitor quality, while also encouraging the recruitment of doctors into primary care. The 24-hour responsibility of GPs was a factor in their high attrition rate. The explanations for this, however, have focused on the pressures that this applied on doctors and their families, and on the difficulties of providing 21st-century quality medicine out of the GP's traditional black bag. Retaining GPs, while ensuring access by co-ops and deputising services alike to medical records, has come to be a vital NHS and ministerial ambition. Some of Titmuss's concerns related to an era when mobility, lifestyles and technology, especially of communications, were utterly different. The challenge that Titmuss would have relished is to adapt the GP-oriented NHS to such changes, without losing its ethos.

What Titmuss achieves in this 1957 lecture is an impressive tour of the insightful sociological studies conducted, at least in the UK, in the decades *after* his death. His review includes insights into practitioner–patient interaction; perceptions of health, illness and ageing; recognition of the effects of new media on expectations of health and freedom from pain; inequalities of patient access and knowledge; issues of medical prestige and what Freidson called "organized autonomy" (Freidson, 1970); and the compartmentalisation of medical knowledge and its impact on patients trying to find their way around the system. In so wide-ranging a review, it is unsurprising that Titmuss does not yet explore some other current preoccupations, including patients' responsibility for their own health (Armstrong, 2002) and concomitant 'patient-induced' illnesses, such as those linked to smoking (where he proved tragically unaware), obesity and car accidents. Titmuss only hints at a need to tackle iatrogenic (hospital or doctor-induced) illness, whether caused by negligence, complacency or the state of medical knowledge. However, his focus on altruism was fed by his belief that a national health service would invite higher standards of staff commitment to care, health promotion and professional collaboration than would apply in a market-driven context. The accusation by his critics of naivety about human motivation is arguably the same as the widespread conservative criticism of all so-called 'command economies' over the past century. But, unlike them, the NHS continues to attract consumer loyalty and popular pride of ownership; in the face of this, it has proved in the past two decades also to be an abiding sacred cow across the British political spectrum.

Tellingly, Titmuss observes that there is a "tendency to attribute all that is thought of as 'good' or 'bad' in medical care to a particular administrative structure and organization". By implication, he casts doubt on the repeated attempts at NHS reorganisation that the service and its million employees have had to withstand in the decades since he wrote. The first of these reorganisations was designed belatedly to unite a tripartite structure into a single health service and to put the GP at its forefront. This was unfinished business to which Titmuss subscribed. He saw the original invidious separation of hospitals, doctors and the public health and welfare services as reflecting only the outcome of conditions negotiated to bring the NHS into existence (Willcocks, 1967; Owen et al, 1968). He does, however, illustrate how medical knowledge combines with professional insecurity to bring about a convergence in patterns of specialisation, as well as the development of comparable professional structures and hierarchies in the UK and the US, notwithstanding the huge differences in financial incentives and the goals, management and funding of care. He criticises these trends in both societies. Crucially, however, he would still be able to claim for today's NHS that its existence *converts private complaints into public responsibilities.* By contrast, approximately 40 million Americans remain substantially outside the remit of any government agency and the reach of quality health care. No less wastefully, although Americans may be "happy with the quality of health care if they can afford it" (Krugman, 2004), this may not translate into a situation in which even the fully insured can optimise their health in the most effective way. Titmuss would still argue that the NHS comes closer to this goal, especially as measured in longevity and infant mortality rates, through a system still oriented towards primary care.

The second chapter provides a similar exploration of what hospitals, Bloom's 'Temples of science' (Bloom, 1965), do to people. It begins by highlighting the same difficulty faced by the generalist lay 'outsider' deputed to manage experts operating in a complex institution or to judge the issues to which they devote their lives. It proceeds to intimate the danger that hospitals tend to "be run in the interests of those working in and for them, rather than in the interests of patients" (see page 135). Like many of Titmuss's preoccupations, these are questions that have no lesser validity today, although, with the added piquancy caused by some high-profile cases of dangerously arrogant incompetence by a few professionals (see, for example, Kennedy Commission, 2001) and by the diverse reactions of government-imposed standards, target setting and other external output measures.

Another concerns patient autonomy and awareness. Pointing to what he politely calls "discourtesies of silence", Titmuss illustrates how people working all the time in an institution may unthinkingly neglect to inform or consult patients passing through their care. He makes the common-sense point that "courtesy and sociability have a therapeutic value", perhaps a foretaste of more recent emphases on the importance of consumer-satisfaction surveys. Anticipating later arguments about inertia and inefficiencies that arise in so large and self-perpetuating an organisation as the NHS, he also highlights how complex institutions, multiplying new complexities within themselves, can, unmonitored, give rise to "waste, misdirected effort and the growth of organizational fetishes" that are impervious to self-correction. These still warrant what Titmuss spent his life doing and promoting, namely "externally-directed critical studies, research and analysis", although organisational change, sometimes argued to be over-frequent in the NHS, has forced constant re-thinking of goals and means. One even wonders whether large bureaucracies, replete with patient, professional and political groupings, whose power and expectations shift like forces in a volcano, inevitably have cyclical clear-outs and whether evidence and research data rival them for influence.

In the third chapter, Titmuss briefly alludes to what he sensed was a canard about health benefits from drugs – the disparity that existed even in 1963 between the proportions of national income consumed by drugs and the conflicting interpretations that are put on this. This is society's economic dilemma. For the individual doctor, especially the GP in the front line, what the emergence of a huge pharmacopoeia has introduced is a patient expectation that a surgery visit will result in a prescription for the latest panacea drug, although moves towards a quasi-market may have changed this to some extent. Titmuss suggests that new drugs often have a short life and that the most ethical thing for a GP may sometimes be to admit to being powerless or even ignorant in the face of a patient's symptoms. But there are strong temptations to succumb to pressure to act decisively. In so doing, a GP may be seeming to comply with a patient's wishes, while expensively enhancing a professional mystique; this may not be a route to benefiting the patient's health. It may even be counter-effective, encouraging a much more consuming dependency; or the aura of professionalism may wear off when the treatment proves ineffective.

This is just one of the ethical conflicts to which Titmuss drew attention. He did so at a time when complex forces meant that personal profit, career advancement, status and prestige, as well as political and social demands and patient expectations, applied conflicting pressures to the precept that 'service is the supreme object of medicine', and made dilemmas harder. This was especially so in societies not operating an NHS model.

One other point about this chapter relates to its originally mistyped title (see Sources on page vi). The growth of minority ethnic populations, and greater awareness of population heterogeneity and the needs and rights of other 'minorities' – women, old people, young mothers, gay people – mean that, had he lived, Titmuss would have had to confront different concerns about inequality and subtler definitions of deprivation. Although he wrote about respecting individual patients, his work lacks attention to particular groups of, for example, Moslem women or old Black migrants, as patients with special needs. However, the ethos which he espouses in the fourth chapter in this section of the book, a talk to the national conference of the 1964 forerunner of today's Age Concern, applies to all people who come into contact with public services. He demands, for them, that services and those who plan them be "concerned with the enlargement, or at least preservation, of the individual's sense of freedom and self-respect". This, he argued, gave all citizens rights to money, housing, health, welfare and dignity as well as to "be eccentric", a personal goal for old age that he, sadly, did not live long enough to illustrate. Even the expression may today seem rather quaint and even ageist. Why cannot anyone be eccentric? Like 'spry', there is a danger in attaching this label mainly to older people.

Towards the end of the time in which Titmuss was writing, the focus of reports on old age, perhaps paralleling later obsessions about immigrants, was on fears of a growing 'burden' on the rest of the population. Projections suggested fast growth in very old populations, and much of the policy debate Titmuss cites was couched in terms of dependency on the working-age population rather than benefits to the society as a whole. This emphasis remains apparent now, albeit with two trends competing: although there has been a growth in healthiness among many older populations, courtesy of better living standards as much as the benefits of health care, some survivors experience longer, later and sometimes multi-symptomatic periods of disability, accompanying increased longevity (Grundy, 2003). The shedding of onion skins of life-threatening illnesses, that previously ruined and extinguished the lives of many manual workers and their families, has revealed new layers of illness, especially of types of debilitating dementia. The title of a World Bank report 10 years ago summarises the tenor of policy concerns: *Averting the old age crisis: Policies to protect the old and promote growth* (International Bank for Reconstruction and Development, 1994), while a more recent title suggests an alternative view: *The imaginary timebomb: Why an ageing population is not a social problem* (Mullan, 2000). There appears to be another cycle in operation here, possibly tracking the economic and employment cycles (Bengtson and Schaie, 1995; Estes et al, 2003).

What would have encouraged Titmuss is the documented tendency, even in 'developing' countries, for mass survival into old age. This challenged some assumptions in the 'burden-thesis' reports he cited in his 1964 talk. Something else that interested Titmuss at the time was changes in the use of family doctor services among old people, which seemed to peak soon after the introduction of the NHS and then slowly decline. Despite a plethora of other data quoted, he could find no clear explanation for this. Although, at the time of his lecture, the term 'carer' as used today was unknown, Titmuss expressed hope that this decline in demand related in some way to a growth in available alternative options under the broad range of self-care, community and informal care (Barker, 1980). In these he included enhanced access to social and welfare services, domiciliary care and the chemist's shop. These all combined with better living standards, transport and health education (Barker, 1985) to add diversity to older people's ways of responding to their needs, although today we are still considering the integration of care services for older people and the range of possible roles of the GP in the promotion and management of community care (Glendinning et al, 2002; Means et al, 2002).

Titmuss would have retained his interest in the links between longevity and social class and in the much better rates of survival into old age among higher social classes (Bartley et al, 1995; Smith, 1996; Dunnell and Dix, 2000). Old age, like other ages, continues to depend, for its quality, on differences from the womb onwards, combined with past behaviour (for example, smoking) and life and employment chances in previous decades. These remain more powerful determinants of health in old age than what the NHS can contribute, however excellent and redistributive its capacities or forceful its National Service Frameworks. The papers in this part of the book show that Titmuss fully realised this limit on the potential of the NHS, but he would have encouraged his successors to remain vigilant in ensuring that it continued to be closely monitored for any ineffectiveness in meeting the goals that he upheld for it. A checklist of questions he might have encouraged workers in the NHS to ask themselves still applies. The following examples apply to patients of all ages and in diverse circumstances:

- How can I best enhance this person's (or population's) health and wellbeing?
- How does what I am doing affect this person's autonomy and self-respect?
- If I were this patient, what would I want in this situation?
- Have I fully consulted the patient (or population) about this intervention (or lack of it)?
- How can we work together to ensure that all patients receive the excellent treatment I am striving to offer this patient?

These are the kinds of questions that stand out in these four examples of Titmuss's approach to the sociology of health care.

Medical behaviour, science and the NHS

Although we can make some quantitative assessment of expressed demand for medical care, this tells us, however, very little about the social and psychological, as distinct from the purely medical and biological, factors which cause demand to be made – or not made. We know at the very least that they are extraordinarily complex; that systems of medicine and popular attitudes to health and disease are the products of particular forms of society and cultural patterns. Sigerist (1945) has traced for us over the centuries the shifting emphasis in attitudes and practice between magic, religion (wherein all disease came from the gods) and rationality. From the anthropologist, we have learnt of the variety of ways in which supernatural sanctions operate to fashion concepts of disease and the behaviour of sick people. "Health practices and health ideas penetrate deeply into the domains of politics, philosophy, etiquette, religion, cosmology and kinship" (Paul, 1955, p 459). Sociologists have shown how the 'discovery of culture' has changed our ideas about the significance of health and disease to the individual in the individual's various roles (Simmons and Wolff, 1954). Psychiatrists have broadened our view of the emotional component in sickness and have given us new ways of looking at the growth of personality and the origins of illness. Even the economists have contributed to the discussion by the emphasis they have laid, in the US, on the 'money-back complex' as a factor in determining demand for medical care and, in Britain, on the 'something-for-nothing-complex' as a factor of demand for medical care under the NHS.

Apart from the central importance of changes in the nature and incidence of disease, we are led to see, therefore, that demand for medical care in modern society depends not only on economic factors, on the distribution of poverty and wealth, but – among other variables – on prevailing concepts of health and disease, and on what we think is expected of us in our various roles by our fellows, in the family, at work, and in all our social relations. To individuals, the sensation of pain or stress is in part compounded by their perception of it, and perception depends on a host of factors. Ultimately, many derive from the significance that death holds in a given culture at a particular time. The more that a society as a whole values success in life and fears death, the higher may be its demand for medical care in some form or other. The more that the individual personality is sensitive and self-conscious about the particular role to play in society, the

123

more demanding may be the perception of what constitutes 'efficient function' or wholeness for that individual and for others.

These considerations are of fundamental importance for any understanding of the role of the doctor and of changes in demand for medical care in modern society. They have to be seen as part of the totality of social change which makes society, in any time dimension, a social process. Two major factors of change (or groups of measurable phenomena) can I think, however, be singled out for closer examination. These, in combination with other factors, have radically changed medical knowledge and its practical application since the beginning of the 20th century.

The first major factor can be shortly described as the invasion of medicine by the natural sciences; in other words, the impact of scientific advances on medical knowledge and practice. Specialisation, or the division of medical labour, is in itself an important by-product of such advances, generating in its turn far-reaching effects on the practice of medicine.

The second major factor is the social organisation of medical skill, techniques and practice; in other words, the accepted and approved channels through which medicine fulfils its purpose, and doctor and patient are brought together. So far as Britain is concerned, the main characteristic of change in this sphere is the growth of state intervention in the provision of medical care services. In the US and other countries, changes in the social organisation of medical care have taken other forms with important, but no doubt in many respects different, effects on the role of the doctor and on demand for medical care.

Although it is possible to visualise these two factors of change as separate, distinctive forces, they are, nevertheless, indisolubly linked. Scientific advances have profoundly influenced the social and administrative organisation of medical care. This is true of both 'private' and 'public' forms of organisation. Conversely, the ways in which medical care services have been organised have influenced the application of science in medical practice. One effect of the interaction of these forces has been to make the doctors more dependent on the natural sciences for the practice of their art and, consequentially, more dependent on society and their fellow doctors for the provision of an organised arrangement of social resources now recognised as essential for the application of modern medicine.

The public, and to a substantial extent the professional, view of medicine and its problems in Britain has been largely dominated by considerations of social organisation and political form (and here I am using 'political' in no narrow parliamentary sense). The introduction of the NHS in 1948 heavily emphasised these considerations. As a political animal, the doctor, like the rest of us, saw the effects of the NHS on the individual and the practice as a more potent and direct influence than the less tangible, accumulative effects of science on medicine. So did the patient. The result has been a strong tendency in recent years to attribute all that is thought of as 'good' or 'bad' in medical care to a particular administrative structure and organisation. The preoccupation with such matters of the government's review of the NHS in 1956 (Guillebaud Committee, 1956) reflects this tendency. Similarly, changes in the role and status of the general practitioner relative to those of the consultant have been ascribed to changes in organisation. In consequence, other factors of change, among which the growth of science in medicine is one of the more powerful, have been neglected by those seeking to understand the role of the doctor in modern society.

$$* * * * *$$

At this point, it seems helpful to give some substance to these generalisations about scientific change. At the risk of being superficial, we may consider a few of the more striking advances. The fact that the so-called basic sciences have, as Ellis (1956, p 813) remarks, "swollen, reproduced as it were by binary fission, and swollen again", has greatly accentuated the problem for medical education. In anatomy, a whole new field of living structure has been opened up in barely 20 years by the study of embryology. Physiology has spread so far and wide that it is not clear what is left at the centre. Rapid advances in knowledge in the fields of chemistry, biochemistry and physics have contributed greatly to the study of disease. Organic chemistry, for instance, has now reached the stage when it can analyse to some extent most constituents of the body. The detection of disease processes, now of strikingly greater importance in general practice, has benefited from advances on this and other fronts. The science of radiotherapy, which has changed to a remarkable extent in a decade or so, had as its starting point the discovery of X-rays by Röntgen as recently as the early 1900s. With the increasing use of radioactive isotopes and of knowledge gleaned from fundamental research into the structure of the atom, medicine is on the verge of a further significant advance in its understanding of the structure of matter and of living processes. The borderline between living and non-living substances has almost disappeared in the virus laboratory.

From the contribution of workers in various disciplines, biochemistry, haematology and others, we now have the medical knowledge which, if applied, could virtually eliminate nutritional disorders, including the nutritionally conditioned deficiencies. All this has happened between Gowland Hopkins' first paper on vitamins in 1912 and the isolation of vitamin B12 in 1948.

Over an even shorter period, immense strides have been made in surgical techniques and skills, largely as a result of scientific advances in the prevention of infection, in the tracking down and identification of bacteria, in methods of blood transfusion, and in the prevention and relief of pain. These developments now allow surgeons to undertake operations with relative safety, to investigate disease and to apply treatments, all of which were hardly thought of in the early 1900s.

Next in significance to the relief of pain, without question a far more powerful and effective psychological weapon in the hands of the doctor today than it ever was, are the astonishing advances in chemotherapy which have occurred since the discovery of prontosil in 1935 and the introduction of penicillin in 1940 (Garrod, 1955). "I doubt," wrote Sir Henry Dale (1950, p 1), "whether the change in the half-century in any department of medicine has been greater or more fundamental than this".

The total effect of this irruption of science into medicine is impressive, not only because of the scale on which it is taking place but because of the speed at which advance succeeds and proliferates further advance. "The pace has accelerated sharply during the past few months," according to a leading article in the *British Medical Journal* (1957, vol i, p 150), in noting the discovery of a whole new series of valuable antibiotics. Once the medical significance of new knowledge in the biological and natural sciences has been grasped, the floodgates between theory and practice in medical care burst wide open. Developments in just a few years read like a story of geometrical progression: they include the elaboration of penicillin (about 50 'dosage forms' now exist), streptomycin, oleandomycin and other antibiotics; the application of nuclear physics; improvements in anaesthesia and thoracic surgery; the treatment of coronary thrombosis with anticoagulants; knowledge of blood compatibility; and the discovery of cortisone and polio vaccines.

Some of the more important additions to medical knowledge and skill within a relatively short span of years, lead us to ask questions about their effects on the practitioners of medicine in their social role as doctors. For convenience, we may consider the effects of these scientific changes in three categories: first, their effects on the division of medical labour; second, their effects on the content and practice of particular medical skills; and, third, their effects on the relationship between doctor and patient.

* * * * *

Every major advance in tested knowledge in the natural sciences has brought with it, when applied to problems of health and disease, a need for specialisation in the acquisition of medical knowledge and skill, in function and in practice. This increasing division of labour, mainly (although not always) based on a scientific rationale instead of, as in the past, an accumulation of empirical experience by the individual practitioner, has resulted in great benefits in the reduction and alleviation of suffering and disease. Scientific medicine thus joins hands with humanitarian medicine in being irrevocably wedded to the idea of progress. Irrespective of race, class or age, mortality must be postponed as long as possible.

In combination, these two factors, science and specialisation, have had within a few decades a profound influence, not only on the practice of medicine and the extent to which its objectives are realisable, but on the established patterns of relationships and behaviour within the profession itself and between the doctor and the patient. Inevitably, attitudes and expectations adopted by the patient and by society as a whole about the doctors and their work have also been influenced. Some of these effects of change have contributed to the solution of old problems, but have simultaneously created new ones. We may briefly consider a few examples as they concern the profession itself and the doctor–patient relationship within the context of the medical care services in Britain.

The rapid growth of specialised skills and functions in medicine has greatly affected medical education. In the US, according to some observers, the "formalization of training programmes for nearly every speciality or subspeciality has created a caste system within medicine" (Peterson et al, 1956). This gives rise to new group solidarities, based on likenesses in skills, functions and prestige. As these separatisms emerge and receive formal sanction in a variety of ways, they tend to foster their own particular loyalties. These specialised loyalties, by the nature of their internal forces, often emphasise, in an exaggerated form, status differences. Pressures then develop for these status ratings to be reflected in greater differentials in pay.

One of the ultimate consequences of these effects of science on medicine is to increase the possibilities of misunderstanding and conflict within the profession. The area of conflict about financial rewards, for instance, expands as one branch of the profession strives to increase its relative advantages while others seek to lessen them. Since 1948, the broad result of this internal professional struggle for status has been that the social distances between different specialists have widened (partly, of course, because of the greater difficulties in the communication of knowledge), while the gulf between the general practitioner and specialists as a body has widened further.

Implicit in the growth of separate interests, divided skills and special loyalties is an increasing fragmentation in responsibility for the treatment of the individual patient. The emphasis shifts from the person to some aspect of the disease. Yet, while science is pushing medicine, theoretically and structurally, in this direction it is, simultaneously and particularly in respect to the application of scientific medicine, pulling in the reverse direction – towards more cooperation, more dependence on other people, more group practice, more team reliance on special skills and functions. These contrary forces help to explain many of the stresses experienced by the NHS today – stresses often wrongly attributed, as we have seen from evidence given earlier, to the administrative organisation of the NHS itself. They also make explicable the great debate in the US on how to allocate fees from the patient for divided responsibilities (Fitts and Fitts, 1955), and what to do about the widespread practice of fee-splitting. These questions of who should send in bills to the patient, at what stage of medical care, for what amounts and on what criteria of ability to pay both for individual items and for the treatment as a whole, inevitably follow from the increasing division of medical labour. Thus, as Davis (1955, pp 26 and 129) observes, in the private sector of medical care in the US, "the economic relations of doctors, patients, and hospitals become an intricate, and sometimes a tangled, skein".

Professional stratification in medicine, the existence of effective superiority and inferiority relationships, has become more pronounced. In the past, according to Sir Heneage Ogilvie, "every practitioner had a consultant's gold-headed cane in his surgery" (*Lancet*, 1952, ii, p 820). This is no longer true; a fact that is not attributable to the NHS! Because those who specialise (who aim to fulfil a restricted determinate function) have a higher status in our society, the general practitioner becomes more conscious of inferior status.

Formerly, the 'specialism' of general practitioners lay in their own personalities. What was charged for was predominantly personal service: the intuitive art of an individual and the personal manner in which it was conveyed to the patient. 'Scientific' medicine, in adding its own particular objective and subjective uncertainties to situations in which more knowledge and more certainty are now expected by patients, has profoundly changed these roles and altered relationships. At the same time as these changes have been under way, we have been witnessing a growth in public esteem of the specialist in all walks of life; the generalist is too attached and indeterminate to be in favour in a world of professionalism and expertise. After the introduction of the NHS in 1948, we can trace a steadily rising tide of complaints from general practitioners about their loss in status and their sense of insecurity.

The advent of the NHS converted private complaints into public complaints. It enfranchised complaint, for the doctor as well as the patient. General practitioners, it was said again, had been reduced to acting as sorters, clerks and mere "disposal agents" (Guillebaud Committee, 1956, p 281). They had lost status; they had been excluded from hospital work; they were afraid of referring maternity cases to consultants for fear of losing them; they were paid much less than consultant staff; they had no merit awards; they were not knighted or honoured; they were no longer family doctors. The NHS was held responsible (Hall, 1956; Jenkins, 1956).

The similarity between these statements and observations about general practice in the US is striking. In their introduction to a study of practice in North Carolina, the authors (Peterson et al, 1956, p 7) write: "In the last few decades a new note has been injected into the practice situation in the United States by the growth of specialization.... The predominance of the specialist organizations has put general practice in a defensive situation and has allocated to it largely negative virtues. The creation of certifying boards in medical specialities has closed many doors to the general physician".

The steady accretion in Britain of all these tangible and intangible changes added to the general practitioners' feelings that they were no longer free agents in medical care; no longer wholly responsible for their patients; in short, they became more conscious of dependent relationships. Yet, at the same time, it was being borne in on them that scientific advances in medicine spelt greater personal responsibilities. The dilemma was most obvious over the choice of drugs. With a phenomenal expansion in the range of choice, the problem of selecting the right drug in the right amount at the right point in the disease process adds to the general practitioner's feelings of insecurity. Some of these drugs are immediately valuable and some are worthless; some are harmless and some are extremely dangerous. In these circumstances, the practitioner can walk insecurely with the times, pushed along perhaps by a greater urge actively to intervene in treating patients, and prescribe the latest and most sophisticated of several hundred new preparations. The practitioners then run the risk of surrendering some responsibility for the care of patients to the pharmaceutical industry. Or they may spurn all the advances in favour of some older remedy which they at least know something about. Nor does the training which most general practitioners have had help them to adjust to change, for it is primarily based on hospital medicine – a very different experience from the average work of the average general practice.

In all these ways, the work of general practitioners has been deeply influenced by the consequences of scientific and technical charge.

* * * * *

Finally, I would make a few comments on the doctor–patient relationship within the context of the changes which I have been discussing. One among the many facets of this relationship which may be singled out is the problem for the doctors of protecting and maintaining the conception of their role as doctors in face of these changes and the fact that they are now seeing a more knowledgeable and articulate body of patients. Although acceptance and submission are still widespread in doctors' surgeries and hospital wards, there would appear to be a tendency for more people to adopt a questioning and critical attitude to medical care. The advertising of drugs, the prestige of science in medicine, the use of television and radio for 'health education', the spread of middle-class attitudes and patterns of behaviour, and a long public health campaign for the early detection and prevention of disease all evoke a more questioning attitude. That is the aim of health education; to make people think about health and disease in a positive way rather than to submit to life 'as it happens'.

Clark-Kennedy (1955, p 619), in writing on "medicine in relation to society", has expressed the view that the attitude of the patient to the doctor has changed considerably in recent years. "He is aware that his doctor now knows relatively much less about medicine as a whole than he did a few years ago." Hence the growing faith in specialists. From what evidence exists, it would seem that this attitude is more pronounced (so far as demand on the NHS is concerned) among middle-class and professional workers. An American study of "cultural components in responses to pain" (Zborowski, 1952, p 27) has shown that the educational background of the patient plays an important role in their attitude to the symptomatic meaning of pain sensation. "The more educated patients are more health-conscious and more aware of pain as a possible symptom of a dangerous disease." Related to these changes and differences in attitudes and expectations of what the doctor can or should do is the growth in Western society of the idea that pain is avoidable.

The role of an ill person has become more formalised, more conscious, more separate and distinctive with the growth of an industrialised, individualistic society. It has, simultaneously, and for many people, made 'good health' a more important and realisable attribute for 'success' in life. The concepts of individual responsibility; the toxic and environmental hazards of industrialisation; the problem of social isolation in the modern world, the decline in religious beliefs, and the need, as Margaret Mead (1952, p 171) has put it, "to make self-consciousness bearable"; all these and other social and psychological factors have a bearing on changes in attitudes to health, disease and the doctor.

This heightened awareness of what medicine has to offer, and which has influenced the doctor–patient relationship, has also affected the responsibilities of the family when sickness occurs. The threshold of tolerance of pain among those who are bound by strong ties of affection is lowered by the knowledge that medical action is possible. Moreover, the more that stress is laid on environmental and psychological factors in child care – on factors that are personally controllable and not predestined – the more may parents be led to feel blameworthy (Senn, 1950). As the power of medicine increases, so does the concept of parental responsibility. The urge to intervene, to do something, to relieve pain in one's child, increases as parents become aware of the potentialities of scientific medicine. What matters here is how situations are perceived and how expectations are formed from different ways of regarding situations. George Mead in his book, *Mind, self and society* (1934), stressed the importance in understanding social behaviour of the self-conditioning of the individual derived from past experience and the expectation of future stimuli. Hardy et al concluded in their book (1952, p 23): "... the culture in which a man finds himself becomes the conditioning influence in the formation of the individual reaction patterns to pain.... A knowledge of group attitudes towards pain is extremely important to an understanding of the individual reaction".

Doctors may react to situations of stress by, for example, emphasising their authoritarian role in the giving and withholding of drugs. Unable to tolerate their own inadequacies, they may become intolerant of inadequacies in their patients.

The old compelling empiricisms in medicine, both in the hospital and in general practice, gave to medicine the atmosphere and tradition of an authoritarian art. Scientific medicine has undermined some of these personal individual authoritarianisms in medicine. It has let into clinical medicine a new spirit of criticism and questioning; it has raised more doubts about the value of bedside observations; it has imposed a different set of self-disciplines on the doctor and, while giving a greater potential freedom for independent thought and action, it has, simultaneously, made the doctor more dependent on other people. The danger is that in the stage through which we are now passing, a new authoritarianism will replace or be superimposed on the old one, partly because of a lack of knowledge of how to use the new scientific instruments, and partly because of the authority that science itself invests in those whose work is scientifically oriented.

Obviously, there are dangers for both doctor and patient alike in this situation transformed by the factors of science and specialisation. Not least among the benefits of the NHS is the fact that we can now see somewhat more clearly the nature of these dangers. There is a danger of medicine becoming a technology (Newman, 1957). There is the problem of medical power in society; a problem which concerns much more of our national life than simply the organisation of medical care. It is, however, beyond my competence to suggest the many checks and balances which might be brought into play to offset these dangers and to correct the imbalance for which science is partly responsible. One at least, I am sure, must be found in the reform of medical education. Another may come in time from the contribution of the sociologist and the social worker to a greater understanding of the dynamics of human relationships. "Medicine," as Pulvertaft (1952, p 839) has said, "can never become fully scientific unless it becomes completely inhuman". The task of the future is to make medicine more 'social' in its application without losing in the process the benefits of science and specialised knowledge.

This, to me, is the fundamental justification for Britain's NHS. It is the prerequisite for an understanding of the problem; the framework through which medicine may more nearly fulfil its honoured purpose; the means by which the freedom of patient and doctor alike may be enlarged.

The hospital and its patients

In depth and range of complexity, the hospital as a social institution has few rivals today. In a study of the hospital, Edward Churchill (1949), writing from the famous Massachusetts General Hospital, said: "The hospital is one of the most complex and dynamic instruments of contemporary society". In Britain, we need to view the hospital in a similar sense – operating within the additional complexities of a nationwide government-financed, centrally-regulated system of administration. No community could hope to succeed with such an enterprise without a large fund of intelligence, and what I like to call 'cultivated commonsense'. The UK has been conspicuously successful in producing administrators with these talents, but such gifts by themselves are not now sufficient when it comes to controlling and administering a hospital service. We must add a wide knowledge of the NHS as a whole, a thorough grasp of the work and functions of all departments of the hospital, and at least a nodding acquaintance with a variety of technical, medical and professional terms. I do not wish to join with those who would make a mystique of administration, but I must say that in my experience most lay members, newly-appointed, of a hospital board or management committee are pretty useless during their first year of office. Often, their sense of inadequacy and the efforts they feel they must make to justify themselves in their new role encourage behaviour round the committee table which is either sentimental or grandiose, or both. I suggest that it is not until perhaps half the three years have gone by that a new member can play a really useful part in hospital government. The Ministry of Health and the regional boards have, I think, over-estimated their ability at spotting talent for hospital management, and, in setting the term of office at three years, under-estimated the time it now takes to acquire a grasp of the complexities of the modern hospital system.

This, however, is but one reflection of the complexities of the hospital world. The central point I wish to make is that we are here faced with one of the most complex of social institutions, an institution which has grown immensely in its complexities and to which we have added – and, indeed, are still doing so every day – new complications as a result of the development of the NHS. Now, in this situation there are, I suggest, three main dangers.

The first danger is that increasing complexity in structure, functions and administration can lead to increasing economic and social costs without a proportional rise in value rendered to the community. Complex institutions and societies carry within themselves a strong tendency to make and multiply new complexities, and each one in itself represents another possibility of waste, misdirected effort and the growth of organisational fetishes. Clearly, the more complex a situation is, the harder it becomes to put one's finger on sources of inefficiency and the fewer chances there are of self-correction or adjustment from within the institution itself. This points to the need, all too little recognised, for externally directed critical studies, research and analysis of the hospital services. No institution, continually in a state of change, constantly subject to the pressure of many vested interests and forces, can hope to remain healthy without criticism. But it is not criticism in quantity that is wanted, or comment of the generalised and often biased type which fills so many of the pages of the Eleventh Report from the Select Committee on Estimates (Session 1950-51, Regional Hospital Boards and Hospital Management Committees, 1951). The need is for informed criticism based on a study of the facts. How necessary the searchlight of investigation and public opinion is to the health of hospitals was first shown by Florence Nightingale who spent so many years of her life in ruthlessly assembling and arranging facts. Even in the last 10 years [1940-50] we have had two examples of the working of this principle: an improvement in hospital food for patients and an improvement in the arrangements for parents to see their sick children in hospitals. The important thing to note here is that both these consequences did not result from any ferment of self-examination in the hospitals themselves or from the professional ranks of nurses and doctors. Broadly speaking, these changes, now accepted as desirable, were the result of pressures from without the hospital. The demand for change came from sources of opinion outside the institution.

The second danger to the hospital and its patients, arising from increasing complexity in the hospital world, is that the ends or aims of hospital work may be obscured by excessive preoccupation with means. Those concerned with policy making and management are increasingly immersed in the details of administration. Each particular tree and, indeed, each particular branch of each tree, becomes more important than the aims of the hospital as a social institution. Boards of Governors and Management Committees devote more of their time to the conditions of work, questions of rewards, difficulties of status and dissatisfaction among the staff, than they do to the needs of the patients. Of course, all these questions are vital to the efficient and harmonious running of a hospital and there must be some system of settling these often difficult issues. But the NHS has added greatly to the volume of administrative work of this kind by the introduction of national uniform scales of reward, hours of work, holidays, superannuation, and so forth. The continual need for the ironing-out of innumerable small injustices and anomalies in the working conditions of members of hospital staffs gives rise to a lot of work and partly accounts for the increase in administrative costs since 1948. Do not think here that I am critical of the need for justice and equity among hospital staffs. The improved pay and conditions of work of nurses and other hospital workers has been one of the great benefits of the NHS. Indeed, one of the major social consequences of the NHS is that it has given not only better conditions but more professional freedom, in the vocational sense of the word, to professional groups working in the hospital. Doctors have no longer to concern themselves with the financial means of the patients; nurses do not have to deal with all the food that patients and their relatives were required to bring into the hospital; almoners no longer have to consider whether this or that patient is a Poor-Law case. An analysis of changes in function among different professional groups would show the extent to which the NHS has led to an enlargement of professional freedom. This is an important gain. Nevertheless, it is wise to remember that all social change on this scale, while solving some problems, invariably creates new ones. One of the new problems is the danger that hospitals may tend increasingly to be run in the interests of those working in and for them, rather than in the interests of the patients. The fundamental purpose of the hospital must not be dimmed by excessive preoccupation with the means.

The history of social institutions offers us many warnings. We need only remember the fate of the monasteries or, nearer in time, the shocking conditions of many children's homes revealed in the Curtis Report of 1946 after the social conscience had been asleep for too many years. Let me quote again from Edward Churchill's (1949) survey of the history of hospitals. Of the changing relationship of the hospital and the medical profession during the 20th century, he writes:

> This blending of the interest of the doctor with the function of the hospital led to a sense of responsibility and ownership.... Society, in turn, has been only too ready to relinquish some of its responsibility and relax its efforts. The doctors are supposed to know what they are doing, and comfort is taken in the attitude that it is impossible for a mere layman to judge of such matters.... This situation has created a disturbing undercurrent of thought that only a few observers appear to notice. Is it well for society, or in the long run, for the profession, that this trend continue? Can a not disinterested profession be entrusted with an agency of society that is becoming more vital today than ever before in history? However sincere the efforts of the doctor to provide the best care for his patients, the fact must be faced that these same efforts provide him with the prestige and comfortable living which he claims. It is

possible that the profession is unconsciously drifting into a dangerous position not wholly unlike that in which the Church found itself before the Reformation.

To Churchill's words, we may add the rider that the advent of the NHS may have arrested this historical trend – or it may not. One thing at least we may be sure of: a social process of this importance, in whatever direction it has been tending since 1948, has not stood still. We have achieved a better or a worse balance of interests; a better or a worse distribution of administrative and executive power.

I come now to the third of my points of danger to the welfare of patients. This is represented by scientific and technological advance. What I have to say relates to the social and psychological welfare of patients in a hospital situation of applied scientific medicine. For a number of reasons, these advances of science into the hospital have made it harder to treat the patient as a person. One reason is that more science has meant more division of labour and, inevitably, of course, more professional fragmentation as specialisms have developed and new groups of workers have banded themselves together in professional groups. An increase in the division of labour means that more people with different functions and skills to perform are brought into contact with the patient. Each separate function to be performed, for out-patient as well as in-patient, involves the sick person in a personal contact with more people – more 'experts' (for that is how they often appear to the patient). All this happens at a time when the patients, sick perhaps in mind as well as in body, with fears and anxieties about themselves and their families, with more questions and uncertainties in a mind disturbed by illness, are less able to cope with the strain of entering into new personal contacts with many strange individuals endowed with all the authority and mystery which surround the hospital and its gift of survival. As most of us know, to feel ill is to feel unadventurous, to want to retreat from life, to have one's fears removed and one's needs met without effort. Physical illness can play queer tricks with our thoughts and our behaviour. This does not mean, as some all too easily suppose, that we are neurotics. In being querulous and ungrateful, demanding and apathetic in turn, we are in fact behaving as ill people. The demands that people make on society are greater when they are ill than when they are well. Yet the advent of science has made it more difficult, in social and psychological terms, for the hospital as part of society to meet these demands. More science means more division of labour and more experts – more of the mysteries of blood counts, X-rays, test-meals, investigations, case-history taking, and so forth. These, in turn, mean more departmentalism and, all too often, more departmental thinking. The fixed person for the fixed duties in a fixed situation is a social menace.

But the departmentalism which stems from a division of labour – from a dividing-up of services rendered to a patient – is given more to silence than to communication. Silence from those in authority, from doctor, sister, nurse, administrator, clerk, technician and so on often means a want of imagination; silence consents to fear among those who have great need for explanation and reassurance.

What is it that patients complain of more than anything else in relation to the hospital? – "No one told me anything ... Nobody asked me ... I don't know". How often one comes across people who have been discharged from hospital, bewildered, still anxious and afraid; disillusioned because the medical magic has not apparently or not yet yielded results, ignorant of what the investigations have shown, what the doctors think, what the treatment has been or is to be, and what the outlook is in terms of life and health.

If one analyses the articles of ex-patients recounting in medical and other journals their hospital experiences, it is interesting how often this theme of the discourtesies of silence recurs. Take, for instance, the story of a mother (published as 'The Iron Curtain in hospital' in the *Lancet*, 1951, vol ii, p 494), who had to go into hospital for gynaecological treatment. The first house-surgeon to examine her did so in complete silence: no greeting, no smile, no sign that there was anyone in the room but himself and the nurse. In the ward, this patient found that one of the biggest worries of some of the other women was whether or not they were to have abdominal operations. None received direct answers from the nurses and none dared ask the houseman who also had examined them in silence. It was the ward sister who told the houseman how the patients were feeling; the patients looked on in silence. "When the morning of the operation came," writes this patient, "and there were ten of us to go, I had some difficulty in discovering where I was on the list. It was quite a new idea to the nurses that it would help to know whether one had to wait all day or whether it was to be got over early." Again, this patient found it was quite unusual for anything to be said before a local anaesthetic was given. Some women were quite shocked because they were dilated under a local anaesthetic without any warning of what was to be done. Drugs were given without inquiry or explanation; examinations were made in silence; infra-red lamps were set going without explanation; people left hospital without explanation. The barrier of silence seemed impenetrable.

Why should all this be so? Why is it not understood that courtesy and sociability have a therapeutic value? Most of us in our own homes know this instinctively, but somehow or other it gets lost in the hospital. Partly, I suppose, it is the effect on people of working and living in a closed institution with rigid social hierarchies and codes of behaviour. The barrier of silence as one element in a general failure to treat the patient as a person has also been created, as I have already said, because of the division of service to the patient resulting from scientific advances in medicine.

Another important consequence of these scientific advances is the greater need for discipline and accuracy in hospital work. Applied science in medical care means precision and accuracy. This, and the knowledge that lives are at stake, calls for a system of rules and regulations governing the performance of duties and the relationships between different groups in the hospital. If the hospital is to fulfil its function without risk to the patient, it is essential that the requests and orders of the doctors should be carried out by the nursing and other staffs with accuracy and completeness. It follows, therefore, that a certain degree of autocratic behaviour by the professional staff is an inevitable characteristic of hospital life. When the doctors are absent, the nursing staff feels that it is deputising for them. Nurses possess, or feel themselves to possess, responsibilities which are in fact greater than are covered by their professional authority, or their knowledge and skill. In situations of this kind – and it happens to many people, administrators, professional workers, and others – there is considerable insecurity if the burden of responsibility is felt to be disproportionate to the knowledge and skill possessed. Inevitably, therefore, as A.T.M. Wilson (1950) has pointed out, these people tend to deal with their insecurity by attempting to limit responsibility and increase efficiency through the formulation of rigid rules and regulations and by developing an authoritative and protective discipline. The barrier of silence is one device employed to maintain authority. We find it so used in many different settings when we look at other institutions where the relationship between the staff and the inmates is not a happy one. It is not a coincidence that the Curtis Committee Report (1946, p 83) on the Care of Children drew attention to the fact that, in some of the most unsatisfactory voluntary institutions, all the children were compelled to eat their meals in silence. This, of course, was not necessary to maintain discipline, any more than many vexatious practices are necessary today in the hospital in order to uphold the authority of the staff in relation to the patients. But certain practices have a habit of lingering on and outliving their usefulness in any type of institutional setting, particularly in institutions like hospitals which are to some extent protected from public criticism, partly because they are concerned with people who are peculiarly dependent, helpless and often inarticulate in the face of authority. The practice of talking between doctors and nurses over their patients still goes on, although it is now known that hearing is the last conscious function to disappear with anaesthesia. Similarly, hearing may remain acute in severe prostrating illness; when the patient may be too weak to move or to speak and may appear unconscious, the hearing function may nevertheless still be active. Again, patients with nephritis are still nursed in blankets in some hospitals, although it has long been known that those suffering from this disease do not sweat and that blanket-nursing is unnecessary. The continuance of the practice is another nursing relic. Even worse, perhaps, is the survival of that automatic rite known as the ward sister's 'purgative round', where all are sometimes treated alike, irrespective of age, condition, previous habits, and so forth. It is an example of what I have earlier called an 'organisational fetish'. It has survived from that great age of the purgative habit – the period at the beginning of the 20th century when the medical profession popularised 'inner cleanliness' and social workers were busy teaching 'outer cleanliness'.

In describing some of the forces which have shaped and are still shaping hospital methods and relationships, I do not wish to leave an impression that the hospital staffs are deliberately callous to their patients. These things are not consciously and deliberately done to worry and distress patients. They are done unthinkingly by people who are devoted to their calling, working unselfishly and for long hours in the interests of the sick. The fact that they can happen is due to many factors. Advances in applied scientific medicine, the growth of specialism, the fragmentation of services rendered to patients, departmental thinking, administrative preoccupation with detail, the absence of critical self-examination arising within the hospital; all these factors, in total, contribute to making the hospital an increasingly complex institution. To these, I think we must add some failure in education and professional training. The sociology of the patients has been neglected – their attitudes, motives, feelings and basic needs. "I sometimes think," said Clark-Kennedy (1950, p 661), "that the unbalanced scientific training which our universities provide is an inadequate education for a man or woman destined to spend his or her life in the practice of the art of medicine".

In earlier times, when the hospital was a simpler institution, and when the natural, intuitive sympathies of doctors, nurses and others had not been overridden by long, specialised courses of training, it was not perhaps necessary to emphasise these elementary needs. Then, because so little was known, there was not the same danger of separating the treatment of the disease – the case – from the treatment of the patient as a person. Diseases divorced from patients are abstractions from reality. Today [1952], as standards have risen and as complexities have increased, the dangers of doing harm to the patient – social and psychological harm and not the physical harm of the 19th century – have increased. The greatest authority of all time on hospital administration foresaw these dangers over a hundred years ago. Florence Nightingale understood that the sick suffer almost as much mental as bodily pain. In her *Notes on nursing*, published in 1859, she wrote, "Apprehension, uncertainty, waiting, expectation, fear of surprise, do a patient more harm than any exertion. Remember he is face to face with his enemy all the time, internally wrestling with him, having long imaginary conversations with him". What remarkable insight for someone who spent most of her life administering and handling facts and figures! "Do not forget," she said, "that patients are shy of asking" – yet how often we forget it today. "It is commonly supposed," she said, "that a nurse is there to save physical exertion. She ought to be there to save (the patient) taking thought." With all her intense preoccupation with means, the design of hospital wards, the planning of hospital space, sanitation, the proper use of record forms and so forth, Florence Nightingale never lost sight of the fundamental needs of the patient. With these in mind, she spent years searching for factual tools by which she might distinguish the efficient from the inefficient, the good from the bad. It was a great achievement, in those days, to employ the comparative method to measure the relative success of different systems of hospital care. Hospitals varied in the quality of their work as much in those days as they do today, and Florence Nightingale's problem (as it is ours today) was to find out why some were good and some were bad, and what could be done about it. Medical and administrative opinion was against her: she was told, in effect, that because of the number of variables to be taken into account, it was impossible to quantify the work of a hospital; different systems and different conditions could not be compared. Nevertheless, in the field of mortality statistics, she succeeded; she proved that it was possible to identify the inefficient hospitals that were doing harm to their patients.

The problem of the hospital in the NHS is fundamentally the same today: the need to know how and why some hospitals are relatively more successful, relatively more efficient, in this or that respect and why others are not. Of course, we recognise that the task is much more complex today. More refined tools than mortality data are needed to evaluate the effects of medical care; more precise instruments of enquiry than costs per occupied bed-day are needed to assess differences in financial and administrative costs. Valuable work is going forward in this field under the auspices of the Nuffield Trust, but there is room for much more thought and study in respect to the methodology of investigation – of how we should tackle these problems in the 20th century. We might, for instance, derive benefit from studying the system of medical audit which has been used for some years by a few leading hospitals in the US. This is a periodical self-appraisal by the entire medical staff of the work performed in the hospital. On the basis of comprehensive and uniform record-keeping, analyses are compiled which show the morbidity and mortality experience of each service and each individual staff member over a period of time. Initial diagnosis and prognosis are compared with the results of hospital treatment, and the results become the basis for self-education and improvement and for the evaluation of new procedures. This problem of the quality of medical care is one of the crucial problems of social medicine in the 20th century. Its importance is increased rather than diminished by the advent of the NHS, by the growing penetration of medicine by science and technology, by the newer complexities of administration, and by all the risks, of which we are often hardly aware, of losing sight of the individual patient.

This is not just a medical matter. The problem of the quality of medical care is in part an administrative problem; in part, a problem of human relations in the hospital; in part, a problem of bringing the hospital as a social institution back into society where it properly belongs and from which it has for too long been isolated. Today, all those who work in the hospital need to care much more about how and why the patient comes; what the person experiences as a patient, and what happens to the patients when they return, as individuals, to society. Unless the hospital approaches its task in this way, it cannot claim to uphold the first principle laid down by Florence Nightingale in her *Notes on hospitals* (1860), when she wrote, "It may seem a strange principle to enunciate as the very first requirement in a hospital that it should do the sick no harm". It is necessary to repeat this principle today. Were Florence Nightingale alive now, she would have been shocked to read Goodall's report in *The Lancet* (1952) concerning cross-infection in hospital wards, slovenly habits and irresponsible behaviour among medical and nursing staffs, and general inertia towards the prevention of infection. She would have seized on the fact that hardly any of the measures to prevent cross-infection recommended by the Medical Research Council were in operation in the 24 wards of eight hospitals studied; that too many trained nurses were still counting dirty linen; that most sluice rooms were in a muddle; that refrigerators contained both milk and pathological specimens; that dressing-bowls, by a time-honoured custom, were boiled for 20 minutes when two would have done; that there was an insufficient sense of responsibility among doctors about the wearing of masks; and that many patients had to stay longer in hospital because of an acquired infection, the average increase of stay per infected patient in three surgical wards being 21 days.

This catalogue of hospital inertia, of primitive customs and habits surviving in an age of scientific medicine, shows once again the need for constant re-examination of hospital activities and administration if the sick are not to be harmed. All these matters to which Goodall draws attention are physical matters, potential physical dangers to the welfare of the patient. That these physical dangers can exist in such alarming fashion today suggests that other and more subtle dangers to the patient, social and psychological dangers, may also be as widespread and prevalent if we did but know. It is the task of each hospital to examine its own heart and to ask itself the kind of questions which Florence Nightingale as a hospital administrator would assuredly have asked had she been alive today – alive to disturb, annoy, worry and help the Ministry of Health and all those concerned with the running of our hospitals.

'Therapeutic' drugs

As a student of medical care looking at therapeutics, I move in a world inhabited more by speculative thought and empirical social studies than by experimental science, quantitative measurement, and controlled trials in the laboratory and the hospital. This means that I shall have to take a broader definition of the word 'drugs' than a scientist might and a wider interpretation of what we mean by 'our society'. I shall also have to draw attention to the fact that human beings do not (and cannot) live by drugs alone.

Although this essay is largely concerned with some of the effects of developments in drug therapy on the doctor–patient relationship, I want, first of all, to say a few words on the question of consumer costs. In most Western countries some 80-90% of the prescriptions written today are for drugs not on the market 10 to 15 years ago (Romano, 1957). In the US, some 300-400 new drugs are now marketed every year (Rozenthal, 1961). In Britain, the national drug bill practically doubled between 1949 and 1956, and led to a series of official inquiries into the costs and problems of prescribing (Ministry of Health, 1959). Under the NHS, there are today approximately some 10,000 possible 'remedies' which may be prescribed.

National expenditure on drugs per head of the population has been rising rapidly in most countries, and particularly in the low-income or 'underdeveloped' countries of the world. There are, of course, difficulties of definition and measurement, and broadly comparable statistics are only available for a small number of countries. These statistics show, however, remarkable differences in national expenditures. Britain, Holland and Denmark appear to be the three low-cost countries, while expenditures in France, Western Germany, the US and Italy are 50-200% higher. Differences of this order are puzzling and cannot be explained without much more research. They are even larger and more difficult to explain when we include a number of low-income countries in Latin America and Africa for which some statistics are available. Considered in terms of the proportion of the national income devoted to drugs, some of these countries are spending more than the richer countries of the West. The cost per person of drugs as a percentage of income per head is three times higher in Venezuela than in Britain. To take another example, Mauritius is today spending a higher proportion of its national income on the products of the pharmaceutical industry than Britain (Titmuss and Abel-Smith, 1961).

The impact of the therapeutic revolution has radically changed in these countries the allocation of scarce resources and the order of social and economic priorities. Relatively more may be spent on drugs and curative medicine; relatively less on food and preventive health measures. There has been an economic as well as an ecological disturbance.

* * * * *

Our addiction to potions and 'medical' remedies is as old as history. Two hundred years ago, Voltaire defined medical treatment as the art of pouring drugs of which one knew nothing into a patient of whom one knew less. It was not until medical therapeutics began to deserve the name of a science in the 1940s that this cynical generalisation lost some of its validity. Even so, most Western-trained physicians practising today in all countries of the world completed their training before the flowering of this scientific revolution in therapeutics.

One problem then for most doctors is how to handle ignorance and uncertainty. Confronted with the patient, they have to deal with this situation in much the same time (on average) as they and their predecessors had before the scientific revolution. There is little evidence for most Western countries that family doctors now spend significantly more time on each patient consultation. Doctors, like members of other 'service' professions, have, of course, always had to perform their role in a large area of uncertainty: about the patient as a person; about the nature of the disease or presumed abnormality; about the effects of therapy. What is different – or what has changed – so far as the doctor is concerned, is the greater relative *awareness* of ignorance in the field of drug therapy. The better the doctor is as a diagnostician (with more effective aids today than 30 years ago), the more likely it will be that awareness of ignorance will be correspondingly increased. More specific diagnosis means more specific therapeutic choices; 'blanket' or 'blunderbuss' treatments will not suffice and will consciously be recognised as inadequate or potentially harmful.

Many more factors operate today than in the past to remind the doctors constantly of their own therapeutic inadequacies: the growing emphasis on post-graduate medical education; pressure from patients in a science-worshipping world; specialisation in skills and functions; the proliferation of medical journals which, on an international count, now number over 7,000; and perhaps most important of all for the family physician, the avalanche of advertising and advice in a variety of forms from the pharmaceutical industry. The makers of drugs are not only telling the doctors what to prescribe and why, but they are also continually telling them indirectly that they do not know. The pharmaceutical industry, like many an academic in the natural and social sciences, is now teaching on the uncertain frontiers of advancing knowledge. The dilemma for the family physicians, unlike the university teachers in other disciplines who can take refuge in some specialised tower, is that it is much harder for them to confess or admit their self-awareness of ignorance. The claims of the profession itself to higher status and greater rewards make confession more difficult. A similar effect operates when systems of paying for medical care appear to require that patients be given something in return for their payment.

The patients' urge to act, to do something about their illness or about the illness of a loved one, to conform to the activity values of society, meets, reinforces and is reinforced by the doctor's urge to fulfil the high expectations invested by society and the profession itself. To expect that anything is possible can lead to trying everything possible. The public behaviour of the pharmaceutical industry, both in relation to the doctor and to the generality of patients, plays the role of a third force in stimulating action. Where are we to look for the countervailing forces which will remind us of the more leisurely 'wisdom of the body'?

* * * * *

Before the scientific explosion, the patient's expectations were of a less *specific* kind. The placebo bottle of medicine certainly had its place (and potentially a much less toxic place) and often formed part of the contract, but it did not dominate the contract or relationship as scientific drugs do today. The bottle of medicine from the doctor, domestic remedies of various kinds and self-medication with cure-all patent medicines all contributed to and often exchanged for one another in the pragmatic 'folk medicine' of the 19th century. In most classes in Western society, consumption of these remedies was on a massive and empirical scale. But the patients of those days, in their relationship with their doctor, looked to a larger extent than patients today for assurance, experience, personality – authoritarian medical wisdom.

Discipline and social control in situations of serious illness found their expression through the personality of the doctors who deployed their personalities as instruments of therapy. They did not consciously have to remember to be what they were. Self-awareness of inadequate personality on their part in those days has its counterpart today in self-awareness of ignorance of scientific therapeutics. Patients can more easily make choices about the former than they can about the latter.

The more that a society as a whole values success in life and fears death, the higher may be its demand for medical care in some form or other. Surrender to consumer behaviour in presumed competitive conditions which are powerfully influenced by exacting standards of 'efficient function' may thus be one consequence of the scientific revolution in therapeutics. It carries with it too the implication, noted by a number of observers, of surrender to the makers of drugs

(Roberts, 1952, p 80). Yet, in another sense, it is the patient who has surrendered by worshipping uncritically at the shrine of science. As Freidson (1961, p 227) concluded in his perceptive analysis of relationships, "... the amount of control that the patient can exercise over his fate in the consulting room is being reduced". The patient is the victim of the assumptions that the individual and society have made about the doctor and of the doctor's inability today to assess scientific competence in medical therapeutics. "Everything has passed beyond his (the patient's) understanding, and he feels like a pawn in the game. This is because medicine, in becoming a science, has been transformed (like thermodynamics or nuclear physics) into something which can only be understood from within, and after long studies" (Péquignot, 1954, p 235).

* * * * *

This speculative 'model' (if it may be so described) of the doctor–patient–drug relationship requires to be qualified and substantiated at many points. It is largely derived from the work of sociological theorists and medical philosophers; no attempt has been made to document it fully from the growing literature on medical sociology. Nor was it thought necessary to present anything in the nature of a cost-benefit analysis in economic and technical terms of the physical and psychological effects of drug therapy.

What is lacking in the research field are concrete and controlled studies which would give precision to these speculative observations, suggesting that the doctor–patient relationship has been profoundly affected by the impact of scientific therapeutics. They are particularly needed to deepen our understanding of the role played in this relationship by three major variables:

(1) *Time and continuity of care.* The problems of knowledge, choice and use of drugs are probably different in degree if not in kind in the case of relatively unfamiliar patients with short-term, episodic illness as compared with relatively familiar patients with long-term illness or disability. Does continuity of care by the family physician act in the patient's interests as a form of social control, as a protection against the feeling of being regarded as an 'object', as a precondition for allowing psychological insights to come into play, and as a stimulus to the doctor not to surrender to ignorance and the latest, perhaps inadequately tested, therapeutic innovation?

(2) *Class and inequality of communication.* Questions of time and continuity in relationships clearly cannot be disassociated from the social, ethnic and educational characteristics of the doctor and the patient. The evidence of such empirical studies as have been attempted suggests that these 'social distance and deference' variables may be quite critical. Their importance has been shown

in mental health studies, in the treatment of tuberculosis, in the impact of a new therapy on diabetes, in partially explaining geographical differences in prescribing behaviour by family physicians in Britain, in experimental social survey research in the US, in studies of teacher–pupil relationships in American and English schools and, most sharply of all, in studies of the impact of Western medicine on primitive cultures. This body of knowledge, accumulating unevenly in various sectors of the behavioural sciences, does show that there are group differences – whether we ascribe them to class, culture, education or language – in respect of the perception and self-diagnosis of need; in respect of the action taken to satisfy need; and in respect of the effectiveness of use of such need-services as are available. [See, for example, the bibliography in Morris, 1964.] Little empirical work has so far been done, however, on the interplay of these dependent variables in relation to drug therapy.

(3) *Systems of organising medical care.* Different ways in which medical care is organised, financed and administered are known to influence the quality and quantity of doctor–patient relationships independently and in association with other variables. Such systems cannot be neutral. Every type of system, private and public, embodies a set of rights and obligations for both doctor and patient. These become part of the doctors' and patients' expectations of each others' role and role performance and, simultaneously, their self-images of expected behaviour. In these situations of doctor–patient expectations, which may coincide or conflict, the modern drug is today playing an increasingly significant part. How significant and with what consequences will depend, inter alia, on the values and goals of different medical care systems.

* * * * *

Lastly, we come to the question of medical ethics and the impact on traditional codes of behaviour of the scientific revolution in therapeutics. If medical care were not controlled (or assumed to be controlled) by some special ethical prescriptions, much of this discussion would be irrelevant. It would have to be conducted in the language of the marketplace, but in all Western societies it is declared that the supreme object of medicine is service and not personal profit. The essence of professional behaviour and the patients' confidence in a profession is thus *predictable service to people*. Predictable, in this context, can be translated as 'truthful'. Practitioners have a fiduciary trust to maintain certain standards predictable to patients. This is the basis of the rule restricting competition, the rule which forbids a physician from treating another physician's patients without their authority. It is, however, the special nature of the relationship which creates the dilemmas for the physician in the field of drug therapy. How can the general practitioner be helped to raise standards of ethical behaviour, faced with the challenge of uncertainty, ignorance, and error in the choice, use and effects of drugs? What are the implications for the doctor's training and education, for the education of patients, for the making of medical-care policy, for the evaluation of new drugs and for the production of drugs?

These are international problems, for the therapeutic revolution has taken place in many parts of the world before the development of professional codes of behaviour. These codes were slow to evolve in the West. The shape and direction they took depended as much on the will of society in general as it did on the policies of the profession itself. Above all, they depended on the growth of the idea of disinterested service. As many witnesses have testified, the advent of science has subjected these codes to serious and widespread stresses (Landis, 1955).

In many countries of Africa, Latin America and the Far East, however, the drug revolution is spreading at an ever-quickening pace and, virtually, in an ethical vacuum. The soil is richly receptive. Traditional cosmologies and attitudes to health and disease readily absorb modern therapeutics. The popularity of the administration of intramuscular injections, for example, with its ritual of aseptic precautions and the apparently magical quality of the act of acupuncture, has been reported by observers in practically every 'underdeveloped' society. It is, moreover, profitable; it enables the doctor to avoid time-consuming human relationships; it does not require the patient to change habits and ways of life, and it thus allows the doctor to contract out of the aspirations of the newly independent nations. Societies which desperately need preventive health practices are being told by Western scientific medicine that they can purchase health passively. Drugs become substitutes for cultural change. Standardised therapeutic procedures substitute for medical humanity, and the pharmaceutical industry and other agencies simultaneously provide "an amazing variety of ancient and ineffective drugs from overseas" (Prentice, 1963).

These are not the only consequences. Drug addiction is growing in Africa. The emergence and rapid spread of drug-resistant organisms in India and many parts of Africa is worsening the problem of control over tuberculosis and other diseases. Pharmacies are owned by doctors (and sometimes financed by the industry) and these sell potentially toxic compounds over the counter on credit terms and on an irregular basis to all comers. One authority concluded that one of the dangers threatening medicine in Africa was the private doctor who was not observing any medical code and was "playing on the credulity of the naïve and superstitious" (Gear, 1960, p 1020).

Two very general propositions emerge from this brief survey. The first is that these scientific advances in drug therapy now need, for their efficacy, stricter professional codes of behaviour – more explicit and comprehensive value-systems of expected norms of medical behaviour derived from professional reference groups.

The second is that the greater the social and cultural differences between the doctor practising Western medicine and the patient, the greater is the need for high standards of professional ethics. The fewer the differences in language, perception, behaviour and modes of life, the easier understanding and treatment becomes, thus reducing the potential power of the doctor over the patient. Their relationship must remain fundamentally unequal, despite, one might add, the Drug Amendments Act of 1962 and the establishment of the voluntary Dunlop Committee in Britain. We have to strive, however, for less inequality. These generalisations apply with added force to countries undergoing rapid social change, detribalisation and urbanisation, with all their concomitant effects in diminishing the sway of fatalism and creating new expectations of health and wellbeing.

Planning for ageing

We are, it seems, all planners now. Harmoniously and ideologically at peace, we are all now to be busy planning community care for older people.

It is not my intention to quarrel with this change in the climate of opinion. As a citizen, looking reflectively at the apparent chaos of activity and non-activity at the town hall or local level, I rather welcome it. As an individual, however, I would like to be sure that, when my time comes, my right to be eccentric in old age will not be eroded by busy, bureaucratic planners. I shall want some rights to some choice of services; not a simple confrontation between, on the one hand, institutional inertia, and, on the other, domiciliary inaction. In other words, I believe that the most important fundamental principle which should guide the planning of services for older people is concerned with the enlargement, or at least the preservation, of the individual's sense of freedom and self-respect. In the world in which we live, by far the largest practical contribution that can be made in applying this principle is to see that many more older people have more spare cash in their pockets, and more in their shopping baskets, and adequate housing to sustain their self-respect.

Planning, if it means anything at all in relation to the social and economic needs of particular groups in society, means the making of decisions about the allocation of resources and claims on resources in the future as well as the present. If we are to plan for older people to have a larger share of the national income, then we are, in effect, planning for others to have less. What we call 'income maintenance', or in more homely terms, pensions, superannuation and national assistance, thus becomes, if this principle of spare money in one's pocket has priority, the most important single area of decision making in planning for ageing. No increase in the quantum of community care for older people can compensate for inadequate income and inadequate housing. We may gain in satisfaction from being busy as community carers but older people will lose in self-respect.

One distinction we can make between the arts of planning and of non-planning (for in this area of social policy both forms of behaviour belong more to art than to science) is in our attitude to facts. If we are to be more intelligent in the formulation of policies and in the administrative provision of services (while accepting that intelligence is not the prerogative of planners), we have to cultivate a greater respect for facts. "Now, what I want is Facts," said Mr Gradgrind, in

Hard times. To look and plan ahead, we require to know more about the dimensions and categories of need and potential need in the future, locally and nationally. To plan and guide wisely, we have also to pay our respects to the past. We have to ask questions about past trends; about where we have come from; about what we have tried to achieve, and with what success.

'Community care' may be a new concept, a new idea, a sweeter-smelling rose, a more promising health and social hybrid, but it has to grow in the soil we have. That soil is composed of some well-known, under-cultivated, but deeply weathered, particles. We can say that we have to work with the existing structure of central, local and health service government (or something very like it), with administrative and executive tools which may be ill-suited for the tasks in hand, with staffs whose training and skills have been neglected in the past, and with little empires of power and professional self-indulgence in local government, central government and voluntary organisations. As G.K. Chesterton once remarked, "God expresses himself in many ways, even by local government". We do not indeed start, as some academic planners sometimes imply, with a clean slate. Reality starts with history.

Obedient to this precept, I want therefore to spend a little time looking back over the past 10 years [about 1954-64]. I begin with some facts about the population of older people just as the Ministry did in its *Ten-year planning report*. These, for obvious statistical reasons, are restricted to England and Wales; to our friends in Scotland and Northern Ireland, I should say that the general results are very similar.

At the end of 1952, the Registrar-General (December 1952) published one of his well-known projections of future populations. He gave estimates for 1962 as well as for longer periods of time ahead. Taking all those aged 65 and over, the population was estimated to increase in the 10 years by virtually one million – to nearly six million (5,939,000) by 1962. These and later estimates provoked much alarm about the social and economic costs of an ageing population. Indeed, the nation experienced in the middle 1950s an almost neurotic and fear-ridden phase; the concept of subsistence was formally abandoned; the Committee on the Economic and Financial Problems of the Provision for Old Age (Cmd 9333, 1954) recommended that the age of retirement be raised to 68 for men and 63 for women, and the Treasury took action to shift part of the current and future costs of pensions from the taxpayer to those who paid flat-rate and regressive national insurance contributions.

How, in the event, have these estimates of 1952 turned out? Summarising the results, we can say that in 1962 we had 337,000 fewer older people than were estimated 10 years earlier, or, roughly, only two thirds of the expected increase. The Registrar-General was closer (or more successful) in estimating the future number of older women than older men; not because, I should add, of any statistical predilection for ladies but due to different mortality trends between the sexes.

The fact that we have substantially fewer older people today than we expected 10 years ago to have is due to higher than expected mortality rates, particularly among men. Death rates among older people have not fallen as much as the 1952 estimates implied. The expectation of life at age 65 (and also 75) among men hardly changed at all in these 10 years; there was only a minute improvement in the figures. Among women, however, the gains were real and relatively striking. At the age of 75, for example, the expectation of life for women rose by over one year, or by 15%, in the space of 10 years.

It is, I suppose, a matter of opinion (and of age) whether this is to be regarded as one of the signal achievements of modern society – or the reverse. Nevertheless, the steadily widening differential between the sexes – especially after the age of 75 – has important implications for social policy. For one thing, it means more widows and longer periods of widowhood. One of the interesting demographic facts today is that, among women, the chance of having a husband by them is nearly as great when they are aged 15-24 as when they are aged 65 and over. According to the Registrar-General's current projections [December 1962] for the next 10 years (to 1972) nearly 80% of the increased population over 75 will be women, most of whom will have been widowed many years earlier.

To return, however, to the figures for the past 10 years [1952-62]. The fact that the number of older people increased more slowly than was expected has meant that more progress in the provision of health and welfare services could be reported than would otherwise have been the case. Take, for example, the services provided by home nurses, which I have always regarded as one of the critical components in community care, particularly for those of advancing years. Although we know surprisingly little from a national point of view about the actual changes in the services performed by home nurses, it is, I understand, generally accepted that about two thirds of their visits are paid to older people.

Between 1952 and 1962, there was an increase in the total number of home nurses (measured in whole-time equivalents) and the proportion per 1,000 population aged over 65 rose by 8%. However, had we had the number of older people estimated in 1952 by the Registrar-General, there would have been virtually no improvement at all. The progress reported, therefore, was due to higher death rates than had been expected.

Apart from population and mortality trends, what other changes have taken place during the last 10 years? To refer again to the work of home nurses, we find that the number of *persons attended* by them fell steadily from 1,177,000 in 1953 to 854,000 in 1962. What does this decline mean? Is there less average need, as the population ages, for the services of the home nurses? Are they becoming more of an adjunct of the general practitioner in giving injections and other medical services for specific groups in the population? It seems that, while the home nurses are on average visiting fewer people (older people), they are making more visits per patient. Are these additional visits in place of calls which general practitioners would otherwise themselves have made? Do they mean an improvement in the quality of service rendered to some people in need at the cost, perhaps, of others in need?

Clearly, we require a sustained series of detailed studies of the actual functioning of the basic domiciliary – or community care – services. To what extent is there in progress a redistribution of roles and functions between different workers in the health and welfare field? If there is, can we say whether this redistribution is in the interests of patients or in the interests of workers, or both? How effective are these services in reality for those who receive them? By concentrating more services on particular patients or clients, is the area of unmet need widening? Questions such as these were raised by Townsend (1964) in his famous book *The last refuge*. What he did by turning the searchlight of precise observation and study on residential institutions now I think requires to be done for the domiciliary health and welfare services.

Any such study would have to pay particular attention to the scope and content of the general practitioner's work. Let me remind you of what the Gillie Report (1963, pp 8-10) on the field of work of the family doctor had to say: "The family doctor is the one member of the profession who can best mobilize and co-ordinate the health and welfare services in the interests of the individual in the community, and of the community in relation to the individual". Earlier in the report, the authors had stated that the family doctor – "the patient's first line of defence in times of illness, disability and distress" – had been, so to speak, at the receiving end of the biological consequences of explosive advances in medical and scientific knowledge during the previous 20 years. "The results in survival of the less physically fit and the aged have added to the scope, but also to the load, of the family doctor's work. This increased load is the central problem in general practice today."

What evidence is there that the family doctor has been playing an increasing part in the care of older people?

With the publication in 1962 of Volume III (*Disease in General Practice*) in the valuable series of studies of general practice by the College of General Practitioners and the General Register Office (1958, 1960, 1962), we are now in a position to assess something of the role of the family doctor in relation to the needs of older people since the introduction of the NHS.

By piecing together the results of these studies and of earlier reports from the Ministry of Health and the General Register Office, we can discern the broad pattern of changing demands by older people on the services of the family doctor for the period 1946-56. We can look, for example, at changes in the medical consultation rates; that is, the yearly number of consultations per person aged over 65.

Before the NHS came in, the combined rate for older men and women was approximately 6.3 per year (1946-47); that is, on average, all those over the age of 65 had 6.3 contacts with their family doctor every year. This was about 50% higher than the medical consultation rate for people of all ages over 16. After the NHS was introduced, the rate for older people rose to about 7 per year (1949-50). Thereafter, it began to fall. In 1955-56, the rate for older men was 5.9 and for older women 6.4. It was then a trifle lower than it had been before the NHS was introduced. Similarly, the medical consultation rates for family doctors for people of all ages also declined and were lower in the middle 1950s than they had been in the first two years of the NHS.

These trends are, on the face of it, surprising and difficult to interpret. They are more puzzling because of the advent of a free family doctor service for all older people and because, during this period, we know that the proportion of over 75s in the population of older people substantially increased; we know that death rates among older people were higher than the Registrar-General had estimated; and we also know from evidence of research carried out by the Social Medicine Research Unit of the Medical Research Council that disability among men aged 61-63 (as measured by sick absence from work for three months or more among men in this age group) steadily increased during the 1950s (Morris, 1964).

It may be, of course, that in recent years the whole complex pattern of *expressed need* for medical and social care by older people has changed, with the advent in various areas of new services, the changing role of out-patients' departments, the greater use of the home nurse for medical or paramedical duties, the rise and rapid spread of the voluntary movement, and other developments. Much of this is, however, conjectural. What we do know is that there has been a large rise in the use by family doctors of privately organised emergency call services in London and other areas and large cities. It is believed today that over one half of all family doctors in London make use of such services and that one privately-run organisation alone accounts for 60,000 consultations a year (*British Medical Journal*, 1962, vol 2, supp 203). The demands that these emergency medical services meet may not be recorded and counted in family doctor consultation rates, and may not be known to the local health and welfare authorities.

In short, what I am suggesting is that some part of expressed demand for medical and social care by older people which formerly was either not made explicit at all or was directly addressed to the family doctor or the local chemist, may now be finding other outlets. If anyone could do all the complicated sums, it might well be shown that compared with 10 years ago [1954], there are today more workers in the broad health and welfare field, public and voluntary, trained and untrained, for older people to talk to; volunteers with meals on wheels, chiropody services, friendly rent collectors, chemists, officials in National Assistance Board offices, older people's clubs, home helps visitors from a great variety of agencies, and so forth. If this were so, it would be an important achievement but we have to remember that less than 5% of older people in the country receive any help from the home help, meals on wheels and home nursing services. To provide a better 'listening and advice' service is surely an essential part of 'community care' for older people, but listening, important though it is in these hurried professional days, is often not enough. Someone has to accept responsibility for action – and often action by others. It is still necessary, therefore, to ask questions about the role of the family doctor in this changing pattern of need and response.

Constructive thinking and planning for the future development of community care, local and national, must rest on knowledge of the present and the immediate past, and an understanding of the processes already in motion affecting the roles, responsibilities and relationships of many workers providing personal services for older people in their own homes and institutions of various kinds. If we wish to support or to change or to do something about the direction of these processes, we must first understand where they are now heading and we must also identify the forces that are propelling them. This approach is particularly needed in the relatively undefined and leaderless field of community care; a field that requires both a lot of generalised workers, public and voluntary, operating from a variety of specialised agencies, and a number of specialised workers operating from generalised and specialised agencies. It is for this reason that I have spent some time looking back at past trends in the family doctor service as it affects older people.

What of the future? First, a few words again about population trends. From the projections of the Registrar-General (1962), we can say that the health and welfare services may expect, *if* these estimates are anywhere near borne out, just over one million more people aged over 65 in the next 10 years. Nearly one third of this additional population is expected to be aged 75 and over; 7% of the increase (nearly all of them women) will be aged 85 and over. Compared with what we actually experienced in the past 10 years, the expected increase in the next 10 years will be substantially greater. In other words, the rate of increase in the provision of services will have to accelerate just to stay where we are today, let alone meet the need, as the Ministry have emphasised, to realise the 'full potential' of community care.

With rising standards of living among some sections of the older population and more geographical mobility in the country generally, we must expect demands for community care to fall much more heavily in some areas than in other others. Geographical differences in demand will be further accentuated as the proportion of over-75s in the total older population increases substantially.

This underlines the point made in the last annual report of the National Corporation for the Care of Old People (1963); attention was there drawn to the "apparent failure of many local authorities to relate their plans to their future estimated population of old people, particularly those over 75". We must expect not only more demand in general for certain old age services but an even greater demand for these services in certain local authority areas. The services and agencies which are likely to be chiefly affected include the following: the general practitioner; the home nurse; the home-help for shopping as well as for housework; the night attendant and the bathing attendant; the use of equipment and special aids from local authorities and voluntary agencies; the laundry service; physiotherapy services; the meals service; and, by no means the least important, the use of hospitals and other institutions increasingly on a daily, weekend, planned holiday and short-term basis to afford temporary relief for hard-pressed relatives and sons and daughters who may themselves be retirement pensioners or nearing retirement age. We can hardly expect in the future quite the same degree of familial devotion from grandchildren and great-grandchildren as is now given by millions of sons and daughters. In any event, we must expect in the next 10 years many more older people (and especially women) aged over 75 who are single or childless, slightly eccentric and unconforming. The proportion may be 25% or even higher (Titmuss, 1954), and the number will not be small. It seems likely that, by 1972, over one million people in the country will have passed their 80th birthday, most of them alone with memories of husbands and of husbands who might have been. They will be the survivors of a period in Britain's history when marriage rates were low (much lower than today); when the rate of emigration of men was substantial; when infant death rates were still high and birth rates were falling, and when millions of young husbands and lovers were killed in the First World War [1914-18]. We shall be facing more of the biological and social consequences of that war in the next 10 years of 'community care'.

These reflections about the nature and dimensions of the challenge confronting the development of community care for older people raise a series of questions concerning the distribution of responsibilities for that development in the future.

It is a much more complicated problem than trying to answer the question: who runs a hospital or who runs a university? There is consequently more danger for the local health and welfare services of situations arising in which the cry is heard, "It is nothing to do with me". The staffing of the services with more workers whose functions are primarily oral and not manual could make the air noisier with this cry. The 'nothing to do with me' syndrome (which has an affinity with a virus called 'functional specialisation') can present itself in situations in which there is (a) ambiguity about the division of responsibility for planning, policy making, and administrative and executive action; (b) ambiguity about who initiates action at the level of individual need and who sees that action is actually taken, and (c) ambiguity about who sees that a series of actions are appropriately coordinated at the right time and in the right sequence.

We may all need scapegoats in these situations of ambiguity but it is no use blaming everything on the Ministry of Health or trying to find the answer by proposing a separate ministry for community care; or proposing major changes in the structure of local government and the NHS; or by calling once again for the reform of medical education, or by seeking to put all the services and all the workers in one building. Changes in all these areas are no doubt necessary but I venture to think that hitherto we have invested too much spiritual capital in structural goals and buildings (in anatomy) and not enough in this matter of the roles, functions and responsibilities of workers in the field of health and welfare. The one study I know of which did not adopt this anatomical view is K.M. Slack's perceptive report *Councils, committees and concern for the old* (1960). It should be required reading for all those who still believe in the myth of a single focal point, a single authority and a simple solution to the problems of developing the public and voluntary services for older people.

'Community care' is much more a matter of people – of staff – and the texture of their relationships than it is of buildings or equipment; it follows, therefore, that we cannot divorce the care of older people from the care of many other dependent groups in the community.

This discussion, essential for the shaping of public opinion, does seem to point to the need for a clearer and more precise definition and allocation of responsibilities over the whole field of the local health and welfare services. It is unsatisfactory for all concerned, including the family doctor, to continue their efforts to improve the services on the assumption that the doctor is willing, able and equipped to undertake this large, idealised and somewhat nebulous role.

What do we really mean when we use such terms as leader, coordinator, mobiliser, director and planner in the context of community care? Let us remember that we do not make progress by substituting one big word for another, nor do we do so by adding to the number of episodic workers infected with the syndrome 'It is nothing to do with me'.

What does seem to me to be essential is a careful and authoritative inquiry which would aim to define, describe and classify the many different components of responsibility. Such an inquiry would have to take account of responsibilities which relate, first, to the *ascertainment and diagnosis* of social and medical need; second, to the *initiation* of action to see that needs are met; and third, to *continuity* of action to see that effective and coordinated use is made of the services available. These components relate to existing needs, expressed and unexpressed, and to the use of existing services of all kinds, domiciliary and institutional, public and voluntary. In a sense, we can speak of them as *individualised* service responsibilities. Next, there is the problem of defining more clearly (and again without expecting too much structural tidiness) the division of responsibilities for the *collective provision* and *planning* of services today and over the next 10 years [up to the mid-1960s]. Between both spheres of activity, the individualised service of need and the provision of resources, there should be well-defined channels of communication which will allow information to flow easily in both directions. Those who service the individual, whether from public or voluntary agencies, should have easy and flexible access to those who administer and plan the services and vice versa. Community care should mean community involvement.

To clarify these somewhat abstract notions, I want to end by asking a few rhetorical and indelicate questions. They are the sort of questions, I think, which a committee of inquiry would have to frame. In terms of relationships, ease of communication between workers, and effective deployment of services, is it functionally better for the family doctor to deal directly with welfare staff or with the medical officer of health? Can the latter (the medical officer of health) defer as easily as welfare staff and social workers to the authority of the family doctor, an authority which derives from the primary responsibility of diagnosing need and initiating action? Is the family doctor equipped, educationally and with the necessary resources, to diagnose social needs and to have this direct relationship with the welfare services? Is the medical officer of health similarly equipped to administer, coordinate and develop services to meet *social* needs, or should these responsibilities be the concern of a social welfare service at local level?

These are but a few of the questions which are raised at the local and personal level. There are others at a different level which involve the distribution of responsibilities for policy making and planning between the Ministry, the local authorities and the hospital authorities. Here again there seems to be a need for a clearer definition of responsibilities.

I will end with a single illustration of this need for a clearer definition of responsibilities but one which seems to me to be critical for the next 10 years of community care. Hospital authorities, when planning ahead for new or extended institutional provision, do so on the fundamental assumption that some other authority is (or will be) responsible for seeing that there will be enough trained staff available. They may estimate their needs for doctors and nurses in the years ahead but they do not themselves take action within their own areas to increase the supply of trained staff. Broadly, this responsibility attaches to the Ministry of Health and other authorities.

When we look at the local health and welfare services, however, the position seems to be very different. Who is responsible for seeing from the national point of view that enough trained staff and training facilities will be available over the next 10 years, or do we assume that 146 different local authorities (and often each department of each authority as well as many voluntary agencies) have somehow or other to take action to see that additional staff are recruited and trained? Have all these 146 10-year plans been drawn up on the assumption that staff will be available, or on some other unstated assumption, or have they been drawn up in the context of the very grave shortages of trained staff that exist today? What can we deduce from adding them all up in a grand national total if we do not know what assumptions have been made about the availability of staff, the trend of population, the extent of unmet and unascertained need, and so forth?

I realise that I have asked a lot of questions and answered very few. My justification is that, if they are valid questions about the future of the health and welfare services, they will stimulate discussion. In any event, I hope that discussion will endorse my plea for an authoritative inquiry into these areas of responsibility for the administration and deployment of the local health and welfare services.

Health, values and social policy

Commentary: Julian Le Grand

One of the many remarkable aspects of the texts by Richard Titmuss in this part of the book is their contemporary relevance. Although written 30 or more years ago, they all deal with issues that resonate today. The behaviour of doctors faced with a conflict between private and public practice (Part 4, Chapter One), the roles of financial incentives and altruism in the welfare state (Part 4, Chapter Two), the dangers of public assistance creating dependency (Part 4, Chapter Three), the desirability or otherwise of consumer choice in welfare (Part 4, Chapter Four), and the middle class capture of the welfare state (Part 4, Chapter Five): Titmuss has insightful discussions of all of these and each is the subject of current debates which could benefit from the participants in those debates reading his contributions. Even at a more detailed level, there are echoes of contemporary controversies: over the ethical issues involved in the recruitment of doctors from the 'Third World', for instance, or the suggestion that economic growth on its own can solve the problems of poverty.

* * * * *

The texts also offer a useful corrective to those who offer simplistic interpretations of Titmuss's views on these issues, among whom I must count myself. For instance, I have argued elsewhere that Titmuss was a principal exponent of what I termed a 'social democratic welfare state': that is, one run by public-spirited altruists or 'knights', who were trusted by society to work for the benefit of the disadvantaged victims of circumstance or 'pawns'. This I contrasted with a neo-liberal vision of welfare: one run by self-interested individuals, or 'knaves', motivated by financial and other market incentives, to provide services to autonomous consumers or 'queens' (Le Grand, 2003). Yet in the article on Mauritius (Part 4, Chapter Three), Titmuss noted that the doctors there were indeed knaves: amassing large fortunes through private practice and corrupt activities in the public sector. He also pointed out that the system of public assistance in place in Mauritius incorporated damaging incentives, encouraging people actively to masquerade as sick and to increase the size of their already over-large families. He was thus perfectly aware of the possibility that trusting professional altruistic motivations to deliver high quality services could be dangerous; he was also aware that the poor were

161

capable of agency (that is, active and responsive behaviour) and would react to incentive structures if the latter were strong enough.

It has to be said that a clear awareness of these issues does not characterise all Titmuss's writings, especially those concerned with welfare states other than Mauritius. However, his reaction to the Mauritian situation suggests that he would have had an understanding of some of the problems that modern British governments face with respect to public services, especially where quality and responsiveness are concerned. But he would have been much less enthusiastic, to say the least, about the ways in which those governments have tried to resolve these problems – especially when the solutions involve relying on market or quasi-market mechanisms. For instance, although, as Part 4, Chapter One indicates, he would have approved of the current Labour government's commitment to the continued public finance of health care and education, he would have been deeply unsympathetic to the ideas of relying on targets, league tables, private providers and competitive mechanisms to drive up the quality of provision in those sectors. His preferred solution – and indeed the one he recommended for Mauritius – would have been through a tightening up of 'professional ethics'. But even here, his ideas would have been applauded by some modern commentators. So, for instance, Colin Crouch in his recent Fabian polemic against what he calls the 'commercialisation' of the public sector in Britain, advocates improved professionalisation as an alternative way of trying to promote greater responsiveness in public services (Crouch, 2003).

In his policy recommendations, Titmuss generally drew attention to the dangers of the use of market-type mechanisms in welfare (Part 4, Chapter Four). However, it could be argued that neither he nor his more recent supporters were always sufficiently aware of the problems with the alternatives to markets and quasi-markets. For instance, consider the issue of respect for clients. Many would argue (as indeed many did in Titmuss's time, although not very often Titmuss himself) that users of public services should be treated with respect: that is, they should not be pawns, but queens. Or, to use a similar but more familiar metaphor, the consumer should be king. Now consider the activities of professionals imbued with the public service ethos, or more generally with the spirit of altruism. Although to undertake an altruistic act may require a compassionate interest for the welfare of the beneficiary of that act, this does not necessarily imply a respect for the person concerned. Indeed, the situation could be rather the reverse: the altruist often feels that he or she is in a superior position to the beneficiary. And feelings of superiority are difficult to reconcile with mutuality of respect. Some knights need pawns, if their knightly impulses are to be properly satisfied.

An interesting illustration of this comes from the work of Hartley Dean, a colleague of mine in Titmuss's old department at the LSE.

Dean explored the attitude of social workers and benefit administrators to the idea that their clients should have welfare 'rights'. He found that, although the social workers and administrators were committed to the public service ethos (and indeed more so than the people they were serving), they felt strongly that, in their dealings with clients, the latter needed to be 'good': that is, cooperative and compliant. Demands based on rights were viewed as threatening (Dean, 2004).

And here markets may have the edge. As philosophers from Adam Smith to G.W.F. Hegel have argued, market relationships can foster mutual respect and counter human impulses to dominate others. A merchant must respect the dignity of his or her customers, or they will turn elsewhere. Similarly, customers must respect the dignity of the merchants from whom they purchase or the merchants will not sell to them. (See Gordon, 1999, for further discussion of the arguments on this issue by Smith, Hegel and other philosophers.) In a quasi-market, where service users or agents appointed to purchase on their behalf have economic power over providers, again providers have to respect users (or at least their agents) and their wants.

The proposition that market or quasi-market systems can encourage mutuality of respect, and indeed other virtues close to Titmuss's heart, such as equity or altruism, is supported by some recent psychological experiments concerning the so-called ultimatum game. In these experiments, one person is given a fixed cash sum, say, £10, and told to split it in some way with another individual. If the other person accepts the proposed division, they both get the share of the money proposed. If he or she rejects it, both get nothing. If both pursued only their self-interest, the outcome would be simple: the first person would offer 1p and the second would accept it. However, the experiments consistently yield quite different outcomes. Even when played on a one-off basis, the acceptors reject what they consider to be unfair offers; either because they suspect that this may happen, or because they themselves have an innate sense of fairness, the proposers tend to make fair offers (Rabin, 1997).

The particularly interesting thing about these experiments is that the results are *not* replicated when they are tried out in non-market societies. Anthropologists have experimented with these games with Peruvian Amazon tribes, Orma tribes in East Africa and Quichua communities in Ecuador. They found that the less market-oriented the society was, the less likely were the experiments' participants to make more generous (or more egalitarian) offers. Thus, out of $100, the Orma, used to trading cattle and work for wages, would offer $44 on average, whereas the subsistence slash-and-burn farmers, who engage in little trade of any kind, would offer $25 on average (Henrich, 2001). Overall, these anthropologists suggest, experience of market transactions may make people fairer or less exploitative when dealing with strangers.

Pure markets have other, damaging, effects, including the generation of inequality and exploitation, if the starting position is not a fair one. However, that may not be the case for the quasi-markets in health care and education that form the basis of current government policy. Individuals do not come to those quasi-markets with their own, unequal resources (the source of poverty and deprivation); rather, the state provides the funding on an egalitarian basis for all. Users, or agents working on their behalf, can then use that funding to ensure that providers respond appropriately to their requirements.

It is often remarked that the problem with state monopolistic systems of public service delivery is the degree of power that they give to providers of services. Arrogant doctors, insensitive teachers, uncaring social workers, overweening bureaucrats – these are the stuff of the standard critique of state-provided services. There often seems to be little mutuality of respect; instead, there is deference and resignation on the one side, and arrogance, indifference or patronisation on the other. In contrast, a case can be made that, appropriately structured, competitive quasi-markets for the delivery of public services may have the moral virtue of encouraging respect for users, in a way that other systems do not. Users can operate as kings or queens, not pawns.

Moreover, the use of quasi-markets does not have to rely on knavish or self-interested motivations. It is true that for most quasi-markets to work effectively, the agents concerned do have to be interested in the financial health of the institution that is providing the service. This is because financial signals are the way in which the messages are transmitted concerning the responsiveness or lack of it for the service concerned. However, this interest need not be entirely or even partly knavish. Providers of the service may have a genuine commitment to the welfare of users, and feel that they themselves, and the institution in which they work, are contributing materially to that welfare. In that case it would be rational for providers to fear that users will be seriously damaged if providers' own financial health or that of the institution suffers; and to expect improvements in user welfare if finances improve. Quasi-market pressures would then operate as effectively as if the providers were knaves and purely self-interested. And the spirit of caring for others, which Richard Titmuss rightly claims is an essential part of the decent society, would be retained.

Indeed, if it is to work in the true interests of users, the quasi-market system has to have this kind of knightly concern. For, as Titmuss's blood donation example shows (Part 4, Chapters One and Two), providers of public services often have superior information to users, especially about the quality and the costs of the service they are providing. They are therefore in a position to exploit that information for their own ends at the expense of the user, if they are so motivated. In some circumstances, this can be overcome when informed agents act on behalf of users, and/or when systems of contracting are in place. But often even expert agents cannot be fully informed, and contracts, however detailed, can never be complete. New developments in incentive contracting may help here, but there is still a long way to go before the models that have been developed are operationally useful. Hence we must rely on some degree of knightliness among providers so that they will not set out to exploit their informational advantage to the detriment of users.

The danger of introducing financial incentives where previously they did not exist is that, as Titmuss argued, they will turn the knight into a knave – or at least allow self-interested motivations to dominate or even suppress altruistic ones. However, this is not an automatic consequence of introducing market reward systems, provided these are properly designed. At the least, they must be arranged so that knightly and knavish incentives do not operate to motivate actions in different directions. More positively, they should be designed in such a way as to be *robust*: that is, so that the same action appeals to both the knight and the knave. This can be achieved by systems that offer personal (or institutional) rewards for activities that are perceived to benefit users, but for which the rewards are not so great as to eliminate any sense of personal sacrifice that is associated with the activity concerned. (For further development of these arguments, see Le Grand, 2003, Chapter 4.)

In short, what are needed are well-designed public policies, ones that do not allow unfettered self-interest to dominate altruistic motivations. And this is a general message that Richard Titmuss – however much he might have disagreed with some current government policies in the UK – would have strongly endorsed.

Choice and the welfare state

For those of us who are still socialists, the development of socialist social policies will represent one of the cardinal tests on which the Labour government will be judged – and sternly judged – in the early 1970s. Economic growth, productivity and change are essential; about this there can be no dispute. But as we – as a society – become richer, shall we become more equal in social, educational and material terms? What does the rise of 'affluence' spell to the values embodied in the notion of social welfare?

The question of who should bear the social and economic costs of change is relevant to the larger issue of the future role of the social services in a more affluent society. First, however, let us remember the general thesis about 'freedom of choice' now being forcefully presented by various schools of 'liberal' economists in Britain, Western Germany and the US – notably in the writings of Friedman (1962) and his followers. Broadly, their argument is that, as large scale industrialised societies get richer, the vast majority of their populations will have incomes and assets large enough to satisfy their own social welfare needs in the private market, without help from the state. They should have the right and the freedom to decide their own individual resource preferences and priorities, and to buy from the private market their own preferred quantities of medical care, education, social security, housing and other services.

Unlike their distinguished predecessors in the 19th century, these economic analysts and politicians do not now condemn such instruments of social policy (in the form of social services) as politically irrelevant or mistaken in the past. They were needed then as temporary, ad hoc political mechanisms to ameliorate and reduce social conflict; to protect the rights of property, and to avoid resort to violence by the dispossessed and the deprived. This contemporary redefinition of the past role of social policy thus represents it as a form of social control, as a temporary, short-term process of state intervention to buttress and legitimate industrial capitalism during its early, faltering but formative years of growth. We are now told that those who in the past were critical of state intervention in the guise of free social services were misguided and short-sighted. The times, the concepts, the working classes and the market have all changed. They have been changed by affluence, by technology and by the development of more sophisticated, anonymous and flexible mechanisms of the market to meet social needs, to enlarge the freedom of consumer choice, and to provide not only more but better quality medical care, education, social security and housing.

In abbreviated form, these are some of the theories of private social policy and consumer choice advanced in Britain (for example, Lees, 1965) and other countries. Like other conceptions of social policy presented in large and all-embracing terms, these theories make a number of basic assumptions about the working of the market, about the nature of social needs, and about the future social and economic characteristics of our societies.

I propose to make more explicit four important assumptions and, in respect of each, to raise some questions and add some comments.

Assumption No 1: That economic growth without the intervention of comprehensive and deliberately redistributive social policies can, by itself alone, solve the problem of poverty

None of the evidence for Britain and the US over the past 20 years [early 1950s to 1970s], during which the average standard of living in real terms rose by 50% or more, supports this assumption. Evidence for Britain has been examined by Abel-Smith and Townsend in their study, *The poor and the poorest* (1965). Had private markets in education, medical care and social security been substituted for public policies during the past 20 years of economic growth, their conclusions, in both absolute and relative terms, as to the extent of poverty in Britain today would, I suggest, have been even more striking.

For the US, the evidence is no less conclusive and can be found in studies by many, including Richard Elman, whose book, *The poorhouse state: The American way of life on public assistance* (1966), provides a grim picture of degradation in the richest country the world has ever known.

Economic growth spelt progress; an evolutionary and inevitable faith that social growth would accompany economic growth. Automatically, therefore, poverty would gracefully succumb to the diffusion of the choices of private market abundance. All this heralded, as Daniel Bell (1961) and others were later to argue, the end of ideological conflict.

One is led to wonder what liberal economists would have said had they had foreknowledge of the growth in American wealth and had they then been asked to comment on the following facts for the year 1966: that one American child in four would be regarded as living in poverty and that three older people in ten would also be living in poverty (Orshansky, 1963); that the US would be moving towards a more unequal distribution of income, wealth and command over resources (Brady, 1965); that many grey areas would have become ghettos; that a nationwide civil rights' challenge of explosive magnitude would have to be faced – a challenge for freedom of choice, for the right to work, for a non-rat-infested home (Cloward and Elman, 1966), for medical care and against stigma (Office of Policy Planning and Research, 1965); that, as a nation, the US would be seriously short of doctors, scientists, teachers, social workers, nurses, welfare aids and professional workers in almost all categories of personal service; and that American agencies would be deliberately recruiting and organising the import of doctors, nurses and other categories of human capital from less affluent nations of the world.

Britain, we should remember, is also relying heavily on the skills of doctors from poorer countries – due in part to the belief among Conservative ministers and leaders of the medical profession that we were in danger of training too many doctors (*The Times*, 11 May 1962), and the belief among liberal economists and sections of the medical profession that Britain was spending too much on the NHS which was in danger of bankrupting the nation.

Guilty as we have been and are in our treatment of doctors from overseas, at least it cannot be said that we are deliberately organising recruitment campaigns in India, Pakistan and other developing countries.

Assumption No 2: That private markets in welfare can solve the problem of discrimination and stigma

This assumption takes us to the centre of all speculations about choice in welfare and the conflict between universalist social services and selective means-tested systems for the poor. It is basically the problem of stigma or 'spoiled identity' in Goffman's (1963) phrase; of felt and experienced discrimination and disapproval on grounds of poverty, ethnic group, class, mental fitness and other criteria of 'bad risks' in all the complex processes of selection–rejection in our societies.

How does the private market in education, social security, industrial injuries insurance, rehabilitation, mental health services and medical care, operating on the basis of ability to pay and profitability, treat poor minority groups? All the evidence, particularly from the US and Canada, suggests that they are categorised as 'bad risks', treated as second-class consumers, and excluded from the middle-class world of welfare. If they are excluded because they cannot pay or are likely to have above average needs – and are offered second-class standards in a refurbished public assistance or panel system – who can blame them if they come to think that they have been discriminated against on grounds of colour and other criteria of rejection? Civil rights legislation in Britain to police the commercial insurance companies, the British United Provident Association and the BMA's Independent Medical Services Ltd would be a poor and ineffective substitute for the NHS.

There is evidence from recently established independent fee-paying medical practices that the 'bad risks' are being excluded and that the chronic sick are being advised to stay (if they can) with the NHS

(Mencher, 1967). They are not offered the choice, although they may be able to pay. Their ability to choose a local doctor under the NHS is being narrowed.

The essential issue here of discrimination is not the problem of choice in private welfare markets for the upper and middle classes but how to channel proportionately more economic and social resources to aid the poor, people with disabilities or learning difficulties, and other minority groups, and to compensate them for bearing part of the costs of other people's progress. We cannot now, just because we are getting richer, disengage ourselves from the fundamental challenge of distributing social rights without stigma; too many unfulfilled expectations have been created and we can no longer fall back on the rationale that our economies are too poor to avoid hurting people. Nor can we solve the problem of discrimination and stigma by recreating Poor Law or panel systems of welfare in the belief that we should thereby be able to concentrate state help on those whose needs are greatest. Separate state systems for the poor, operating in the context of powerful private welfare markets, tend to become poor standard systems. In so far as they are able to recruit at all for education, medical care and other services, they tend to recruit the worst rather than the best teachers, doctors, nurses, administrators and other categories of staff upon whom the quality of service so much depends. And if the quality of personal service is low, there will be less freedom of choice and more felt discrimination.

Assumption No 3: That private markets in welfare would offer consumers more choice

The growth of private markets in medical care, education and other welfare services, based on ability to pay and not on criteria of need, has the effect of limiting and narrowing choice for those who depend on or who prefer to use the public services.

But let us be more specific, remembering that the essential question is: *whose* freedom of choice? Let us consider this question of choice in the one field – private pension schemes – where the insurance market already operates to a substantial extent and where the philosophy of "free pensions for free men" holds sway (Seldon, 1957). It is, for example, maintained by the insurance industry that private schemes "are arrangements made voluntarily by individual employers with their own workers" (Life Offices' Association, 1957, p 3), that they are tailor made and shaped to meet individual (consumer) requirements. This is, par excellence, the model of consumer choice in the private welfare market.

What are the facts? For the vast majority of workers covered by private schemes, there is no choice. Private schemes are compulsory. Workers are not offered the choice of deferred pay or higher wages, funded schemes or pay-as-you-go schemes. They are not asked to choose between contributory or non-contributory schemes; between flat-rate systems or earnings-related systems. Despite consumer evidence of a widespread wish for the provision of widows' benefits, employees are not asked to choose. There is virtually no consultation with employees or their representatives. They have no control whatsoever over the investment of funds in the hands of private insurance companies and, most important of all, they are rarely offered on redundancy or if they freely wish to change their jobs the choice of full preservation of pension rights (Ministry of Labour, 1966).

These issues of transferability and the full preservation of pension rights underline strongly the urgency and importance of the government's review of social security. We have now been talking for many years about the need for freedom of industrial movement, full transferability, and adequate, value-protected pensions as 'of right' in old age; it is time the government's proposals were made known.

Assumption No 4: That social services in kind, particularly medical care, have no characteristics which differentiate them from goods in the private market

I propose to consider this last assumption in relation to medical care, and to pursue a little more intensively some of the central issues which I raised in 'Ethics and economics of medical care' (1968b). This was written in response to the thesis advanced by certain 'liberal' economists in Britain and the US who, after applying neo-classical economic theory to Western type systems of medical care, concluded that "medical care would appear to have no characteristics which differentiate it sharply from other goods in the market" (Lees, 1965, pp 37-9 and 86-7). It should, therefore, be treated as a personal consumption good indistinguishable in principle from other goods. Consequently, and in terms of political action, private markets in medical care should be substituted for public markets. In support of this conclusion it is argued that the "delicate, anonymous, continuous and pervasive" mechanism of the private market (ibid, p 64) not only makes more consumer choice possible but provides better services for a more discriminating public. Choice stimulates discrimination which, in turn, enlarges choice.

This thesis is usually presented as applying universally and in terms of the past as well as the present. It is presumed to apply to contemporary India and Tanzania as well as 19th-century Britain. It is, therefore, as a theoretical construct 'culture-free'. It is also said to be value-free. Medical care is a utility and all utilities are good things. But, as we cannot measure the satisfactions of utilities – or compare individual satisfactions derived from different utilities – we should rely on 'revealed preferences'. Observable market behaviour will show what an individual chooses. Preference is what individuals prefer; no collective value judgment is consequently said to be involved.

In applying this body of doctrine to medical care, we have to consider a large number of characteristics (or factors) which may or may not be said to differentiate medical care from personal consumption of goods in the market. I want to concentrate discussion on two of these factors, chiefly because I believe that one of them is central to the whole debate about medical care, and because both of them tend to be either ignored or treated superficially by most writers on the subject. Broadly, they centre around the problems of uncertainty and unpredictability in medical care, and, second, the difficulty, in theory as well as in practice, of treating medical care as a conceptual entity.

Consider first the problems of uncertainty which confront the consumer of medical care. Then contrast them with the problems of the consumer of, say, cars; there is clearly a risk to life in both situations, if wrong choices are made. It is argued, for example, by Lees (1965, p 87) and others that the market for consumer durables is affected both by unpredictability of personal demand and consumer ignorance about needs. The more significant differentiating characters in the area of medical care would appear to be as follows (although this is by no means an exhaustive list):

(1) Many consumers do not desire medical care.
(2) Many consumers do not know they need medical care.
(3) Consumers who want medical care do not know in advance how much medical care they need and what it will cost.
(4) Consumers do not know and can rarely estimate in advance what particular categories of medical care they are purchasing (such as surgical procedures, diagnostic tests, drugs, and so on).
(5) Consumers can seldom learn from experience of previous episodes of medical care consumption (not only do illnesses, or 'needs', vary greatly but utility variability in medical care is generally far greater than is the case with consumer durables).
(6) Most consumers cannot assess the value of medical care (before, during or after consumption) as an independent variable. They cannot be sure, therefore, whether they have received 'good' or 'bad' medical care. Moreover, the timescale needed for assessment may be the total life duration.
(7) Most consumers of medical care enter the doctor–patient relationship on an unequal basis; they believe that the doctor or surgeon knows best. Unlike market relationships in the case of consumer durables, they know that this special inequality in knowledge and techniques cannot for all practical purposes be reversed.

(8) Medical care can seldom be returned to the seller, exchanged for durable goods or discarded. For many people, the consequences of consuming medical care are irreversible.

(9) Medical care knowledge is not at present a marketable advertised commodity, nor can consumers exchange comparable valid information about the consumption of 'good' or 'bad' medical care.

(10) Consumers of medical care experience greater difficulties in changing their minds in the course of consuming care than do consumers of durable goods.

(11) Consumers of medical care may, knowingly or unknowingly, take part in or be the subject of research, teaching and controlled experiments which may affect the outcome.

(12) The concept of 'normal' or 'average' economic behaviour on the part of adult consumers, built into private enterprise medical care models, cannot be applied automatically to people with mental health problems, disabilities or other special needs, and other categories of consumer-patients.

(13) Similarly, this concept of 'normal' behaviour cannot be applied automatically to populations from non-Western cultures, and different beliefs and value systems.

These thirteen characteristics are indicative of the many subtle aspects of uncertainty and unpredictability which pervade modern medical care systems. "I hold", wrote Professor K.J. Arrow, in an article entitled 'Uncertainty and the welfare economics of medical care', in the *American Economic Review* (vol 53, no 5, December 1963), "that virtually all the special features of this (medical care) industry, in fact, stem from the prevalence of uncertainty".

To grasp fully the significance of these differentiating characteristics, each one of them should be contrasted with the situation of the consumer of cars or other consumption goods – an exercise which I cheerfully leave to the reader.

I turn now to my second set of questions. Many economists who attempt to apply theories and construct models in this particular area conduct their analyses on the assumption that 'medical care' is (or can be treated as) an entity. Historically, perhaps, this may once have been marginally valid when it consisted almost wholly of the personal doctor–patient relationship. Medical care, we would now say, was more a matter 50 years ago of spontaneous biological response or random chance.

Science, technology and economic growth have, however, transformed medical care into a group process; a matter of the organised application of an immense range of specialised skills, techniques, resources and systems. If, therefore, we now wish to examine medical care from the standpoint of economic theory, we need to break down this vague and generalised concept 'medical care' into precise and distinctive components.

To illustrate the importance of doing so let us consider one example: probably one of the more critical components in curative medicine today, namely, the procurement, processing, matching, distribution, financing and transfusion of whole human blood. Is human blood a consumption good?

The gift of blood

In Alexander Solzhenitsyn's novel *Cancer ward* (1969), Shulubin is talking to Kostoglotov:

> "We have to show the world a society in which all relationships, fundamental principles and laws flow directly from moral ethics, and from them *alone*. Ethical demands would determine all calculations: how to bring up children, what to prepare them for, to what purpose the work of grown-ups should be directed, and how their leisure should be occupied. As for scientific research, it should only be conducted where it doesn't damage ethical morality, in the first instance where it doesn't damage the researchers themselves."

Kostoglotov then raises questions.

> "There has to be an economy after all doesn't there? That comes before everything else." "Does it?" said Shulubin. "That depends. For example, Vladimir Solovyov argues rather convincingly that an economy could and should be built on an ethical basis."

> "What's this? Ethics first and economics afterwards?" Kostoglotov looked bewildered.

The questions raised by Solzhenitsyn could as well be directed at social policy institutions. What, for example, are the connections between what we in Britain conventionally call the 'social services' and the role of altruism in modern industrial societies? And have we a convenient model for studying such relationships? Blood as a living tissue and as a bond that links all men and women so closely that differences of colour, religious belief and cultural heritage are insignificant beside it, may now constitute in Western societies one of the ultimate tests of where the 'social' begins and the 'economic' ends.

* * * * *

The transfer of blood and blood derivatives from one human being to another represents one of the greatest therapeutic instruments in the hands of modern medicine. But these developments have set in train social, economic and ethical consequences which present society with issues of profound importance.

The demand for blood and blood products is increasing all over the world. In high-income countries, in particular, the rate of growth in demand has been rising so rapidly that shortages have begun to appear. In all Western countries, demand is growing faster than rates of growth in the population aged 18-65 from whom donors are drawn. And, despite a massive research effort in the US to find alternatives, there is often no substitute for human blood.

Many factors are responsible for this increase in demand. Some surgical procedures call for massive transfusions of blood (as many as 60 donations may be needed for a single open-heart operation and, in one American heart-transplant case, over 300 pints of blood were used); artificial kidneys require substantial volumes of blood and developments in organ transplants could create immense additional demands. Furthermore, more routine surgery is now used more frequently and is made available to a larger proportion of the population than formerly. A more violent or accident-prone world insistently demands more blood for road casualties and war injuries.

In 1968, more than 300,000 pints of blood were shipped from the US and elsewhere to treat victims of the Vietnam War.

There seems to be no predictable limit to the demand for blood supplies, especially when one remembers the as-yet unmet needs for surgical and medical treatment.

* * * * *

On the biological, technical and administrative side, three factors limit the supply of blood.

Only about half a population is medically eligible to donate blood. Furthermore, the amount any one person can give in a year is restricted – two donations in the British National Blood Transfusion Service (probably the lowest limit and the most rigorous standard in the world); five in the US, a minimum often exceeded by paid donors, commercial blood banks and pharmaceutical companies, using techniques such as plasmapheresis; in Japan, where 90% of blood is bought and sold, the standard is even lower. These differences can be analysed as a process of redistribution of life chances in terms of age, sex, social class, income, ethnic group, and so on.

Human blood deteriorates after three weeks in the refrigerator and this perishability presents great technical and administrative problems to those running transfusion services. But it does mean that, by measuring wastage (that is, the amount of blood that has to be thrown away), the efficiencies of different blood collection and distribution systems can be compared.

Blood can be more deadly than any drug. Quite apart from the problems of cross-matching, storage, labelling, and so on, there are serious risks of disease transmission and other hazards. In Western countries, a major hazard is serum hepatitis transmitted from carrier donor to susceptible patient. Since carriers cannot yet be reliably detected, the patient becomes the laboratory for testing 'the gift'. Donors, therefore, have to be screened every time they come to give blood, and the donor's truthfulness in answering questions about health, medical history and drug habits becomes vital. Upon the honesty of the donors depends the life of the recipients of their blood. In this context, we need to ask what conditions and arrangements permit and encourage maximum truthfulness on the part of the donors. Can honesty be pursued, regardless of the donor's motives for giving blood? What systems, structures and social policies encourage honesty or discourage and destroy voluntary and truthful gift relationships?

* * * * *

To give or not to give, to lend, repay, or even to buy and sell blood are choices which lead us, if we are to understand these transactions in the context of any society, to the fundamentals of social and economic life.

The forms and functions of giving embody moral, social, psychological, religious, legal and æsthetic ideas. They may reflect, sustain, strengthen or loosen the cultural bonds of the group, large or small. They may inspire the worst excesses of war and tribalism or the tolerances of community.

Customs and practices of non-economic giving – unilateral and multilateral society transfers – thus may tell us much, as Marcel Mauss (1954) so sensitively demonstrated in his book *The Gift*, about the texture of personal and group relationships in different cultures. In some societies, past and present, gifts aim to buy peace; to express affection, regard or loyalty; to unify the group; to fulfil a contractual set of obligations and rights; to function as acts of penitence, shame or degradation; and to symbolise many other human sentiments. When one reads the work of anthropologists and sociologists, such as Mauss and Lévi-Strauss (1969), who have studied the social functions of giving, a number of themes relevant to any attempt to delineate a typology of blood-donors may be discerned.

From these readings and from statistics for different countries, a spectrum of blood-donor types can be constructed. At one extreme is the paid donor who sells his blood for what the market will bear: some are semi-salaried, some are long-term prisoner volunteers; some are organised in blood trade unions. As a market transaction, information that might have a bearing on the quality of the blood is withheld if possible from the buyer, since such information could affect the sale of the blood. Thus, in the US, blood-group identification cards are loaned, at a price, to other sellers, and blood is illegally mislabelled and updated, and other devices are used which make it very difficult to screen out drug addicts, alcoholics and hepatitis carriers, and so on. [Commentaries in the 1997 edition of *The gift relationships* refer to other more recent issues, such as HIV and Aids.]

At the other extreme is the voluntary, unpaid donor. This type is the closest approximation in social reality to the abstract idea of a 'free human gift'. There are no tangible immediate rewards, monetary or non-monetary; there are no penalties; and donors know that their gifts are for unnamed strangers, without distinction of age, sex, medical illness, income, class, religion or ethnic group. No donor type can be characterised by complete disinterested spontaneous altruism. There must be some sense of obligation, approval and interest; some awareness of the need for the gift; some expectation that a return gift may be needed and received at some future date. But the unpaid donation of blood is an act of free will: there is no formal contract, legal bond, power situation; no sense of shame or guilt; no money and no explicit guarantee of, or wish for, reward or return gift.

Almost all the 1.5 million registered donors in Britain and donors in some systems of European countries fall into this category. An analysis of blood-donor motives suggests that the main reason people give blood is most commonly a general desire to help people; almost a third of the British donors studied said that their gift was in response to an appeal for blood; 7% said that it was to repay a transfusion given to someone they knew.

By contrast, in the US, less than 10% of supplies come from the voluntary community donor. Proportionately more and more blood is being supplied by the poor, the unskilled, the unemployed, and other low-income groups, and with the rise in plasmapheresis, there is emerging a new class of exploited high blood yielders. Redistribution in terms of 'the gift of blood and blood products' from the poor to the rich seems to be one of the dominant effects of the American blood-banking system.

* * * * *

When we compare the commercial blood-bank, such as that found in the US, with the voluntary system functioning as an integral part of the NHS in Britain, we find that the commercial blood-bank fails on each of four counts: economic efficiency, administrative efficiency, price and quality. Commercial blood-bank systems waste blood, and shortages, acute and chronic, characterise the demand-and-supply position. Administratively, there is more paperwork and greater computing and accounting overheads. The cost per unit is some five to ten times higher in the US. And, as judged by statistics for post-transfusion hepatitis, the risk of transfusing contaminated blood is greater if the blood is obtained from a commercial source.

Paradoxically — or so it may seem to some — the more

commercialised blood-distribution becomes (and hence more wasteful, inefficient and dangerous), the more will the gross national product be inflated. In part, and quite simply, this is the consequence of statistically 'transferring' an unpaid service (voluntary donors, voluntary workers in the service, unpaid time), with much lower external costs, to a monetary and measurable paid activity, involving more costly externalities. Similar effects on the gross national product would ensue if housewives were paid for housework or childless married couples were financially rewarded for adopting children or if hospital patients cooperating for teaching purposes charged medical students. The gross national product is also inflated when commercial markets accelerate 'blood obsolescence'; the waste is counted because someone has paid for it.

What *The Economist* described in its 1969 survey of the American economy as the great 'efficiency gap' between that country and Britain clearly does not apply to the distribution of human blood. The voluntary, socialised system in Britain is economically, professionally, administratively and qualitatively more efficient than the mixed, commercialised and individualistic American system.

Another myth, the Paretian myth of consumer sovereignty, has also to be shattered. In the commercial blood market, consumers are not king. They have less freedom of choice to live unharmed; little choice in determining price; are more subject to scarcity, are less free from bureaucratisation; have fewer opportunities to express altruism; and exercise fewer checks and controls in relation to consumption, quality and external costs. Far from being sovereign, they are often exploited.

What also emerges from this case study is the significance of the externalities (the values and disvalues external to, but created by, blood-distribution systems treated as entities) and the multiplier effects of such externalities on what we can only call 'the quality of life'. At one end of the spectrum of externalities is the individual affected by hepatitis; at the other end, the market behaviour of economically rich societies seeking to import blood from other societies who are thought to be too poor and economically decadent to pay their own blood donors.

* * * * *

We started with blood as a model for examining how altruism and social policy might work together in a modern industrial society. We might equally have chosen eye banks, patients as teaching material, fostering, or even the whole concept of the community-based distribution of welfare to those in need. All these involve in some degree a gift relationship. The example chosen suggests, first, that gift exchange of a non-qualifiable nature has more important functions in a complex society than the writings of Lévi-Strauss and others might indicate. Second, the application of scientific and technological developments in such societies is further accelerating the spread of such complexity and has increased, rather than decreased, the scientific as well as the social need for such relationships. Third, for these and many other reasons, modern societies require more rather than less freedom of choice for the expression of altruism in the daily life of all social groups. This requirement can be argued for on social and ethical grounds, but, as we have seen for blood donors, it can also be argued for on scientific and economic criteria.

I believe that it is a responsibility of government, acting, for example, through social policy, to weaken market forces which put people in positions where they have little opportunity to make moral choices or to behave altruistically if they wish to do so. The voluntary blood-donor system is a practical example of a fellowship relationship operating on an institutional basis, in this instance the NHS. It shows how social policy decisions can foster such relationships between free and equal individuals. If we accept that people have a social and biological need to help, then they should not be denied the chance to express this need by entering into a gift relationship.

* * * * *

When one has spent – or mis-spent – substantial fractions of many years in gathering materials for a study and has eventually seen the results published in book form, one is strongly conscious of a need to forget; at the very least there is a wish not to live in repetitious ways. An ancient Arab proverb, possibly relevant here, runs something like this: the word you have spoken is your master; the word you have not spoken is your slave. And so it is with my book *The gift relationship* which I sub-titled *From human blood to social policy*.

I would like to take this opportunity to express again my gratitude to those who educated a lay person (both orally and in writing) in many of the scientific and technical aspects of blood and blood products, and their procurement, processing, distribution, use, misuse, benefit and harm. I would also now wish to apologise to the Scottish Blood Transfusion Services for not including them in my field studies and in the questionnaire enquiry I undertook of the characteristics and motivations of 3,813 blood donors.

Since the book was published, I have received hundreds of letters from many parts of the world from individuals who have contracted serum hepatitis following blood transfusions; masses of additional statistical material about blood donor (or supplier) numbers and characteristics – especially from the US, the USSR [sic] and India, and much interesting testimony ranging from reports on the British National Blood Transfusion Services being printed in Washington's *Congressional Record* to requests from the State Central Scientific Medical Library (International Book Exchange Section) in Moscow for free copies of the book because of an inability among haematologists in the Soviet Union [sic] to obtain foreign exchange to buy such apparently unscientific publications (a request I gladly acceded to).

From this new material, I have selected a few facts to report. Despite developments in methods and techniques of plasma-fractionation, component therapy, storage, computer programs and so forth, the demand for the supply of whole blood continues to increase all over the world. Apart from rising medical and surgical demands, a more ultra-violent, nationalistic, overcrowded and accident-prone world needs more donor blood if death is to be delayed and disability prevented. From the evidence I have received, it seems that there is a more widespread awareness among responsible authorities of shortages of supplies, chronic and acute, in the US, Japan, South Africa, Sweden, East Germany, the Soviet Union and other countries.

For example, it appears that I underestimated in my book the number of units of blood obtained in the US from various groups I classified (in an eight-fold typology of donors and suppliers) as 'captive donors', paid and unpaid. More use is being made of prisoners (partly because, statistically, more crimes are being committed and there are more prisoners). It seems that this trend has had the effect of lowering the proportionate share in the US of blood supplies from voluntary and other categories of donors in relation to demand. Or it could mean that proportionately more whole blood is being wasted through outdating. But the statistics are inadequate to check these interpretations.

In other countries with different political and economic systems, more inducements and privileges are being offered to popularise and attract donors and suppliers. In some of the Republics of the Soviet Union [sic], those donating blood are given preferences in service at trading establishments, cinemas, postal and other public services. In the German Democratic Republic [sic], where 75-80% of all donors are paid (a higher proportion than in the Soviet Union), similar preferences are being given to those who volunteer to give blood without a direct cash payment.

My main impression in studying this new and additional material is that, in many modern industrialised societies, blood transfusion agencies are finding it harder to attract and recruit the voluntary donor, and, perhaps even more important, to maintain repeated and continuous contributions from such donors. Given the hard facts of rising demands, the changing pattern of seasonal, emergency and geographical needs for whole blood of different groups, and other medical and social variables, it is becoming clearer to those responsible for organising recruitment programmes that effective transfusion services cannot be run on the basis of dramatic and 'crises' appeals to transient or sporadic givers or suppliers of blood.

This was one of the lessons I learnt, aided by the computer, from my study of the National Blood Transfusion Service in England. The 3,616 donors who had all given at least one previous donation had contributed over more than 15 years of giving, a total of 43,391 pints. Of this total, 7% had come from relatively new donors (1 to 4 pints), 34% from those with a record of 5-14 previous donations, 34% from those with 15-29 previous donations and 25% from those who had given over 30 previous donations. What surprised me – although, perhaps, it should not have done so – was that the pattern of giving was broadly the same for women as for men. Both sexes exhibited these characteristics of regularity, reliability and consistency in their voluntary contributions.

What intrigued me when I embarked on this survey was the absence of any collected national data on the social and demographic characteristics of some 1.5 million blood donors in Britain. The French and the Belgians were worried because they had an ageing donor population and were not recruiting the young. The Swedes were worried because, having institutionalised a cash payment (although, unlike the Americans, direct to hospitals and not through commercial blood banks), they found they were relying too heavily on the transient young and such categories as students to whom a relatively small cash payment was a temporary inducement. With rising standards of living, rising demands for blood supplies and a fall in the real value of the cash inducement, was there not in prospect a crisis for the Swedish Blood Transfusion Services? In South Africa, the authorities were worried because they were failing to recruit donors from the Bantu and Coloured populations. Increasingly, there was in operation a system of redistribution of blood supplies from white people to black people in order to maintain supplies to the hospitals.

Since so little was known in most of these countries, I embarked on organising and collecting a mass of statistics about numbers, types, characteristics and trends. Some part of this material was published in the book, but because of the voluminous nature of the response, much of the study is focused on a comparison of the pluralised American system and the national voluntary system in Britain.

These studies, national and international, were based on evidence relating chiefly to the years 1965-69. Since then, many economic, social, technical and scientific developments have taken place. Moreover, large-scale unemployment has increased in Britain, the US, Canada and other countries and other divisive forces have been at work which may conceivably have affected donor-supplier motivations and patterns of demand and supply.

Whether or not they have done so, I do not know. I remain convinced, however, that the voluntary system must be sustained in Britain and with it the principles of regularity and consistency in relationships between the transfusion service and its donors.

Medical ethics and social change in developing societies

I have long been interested both in the historical development of systems of medical care and in the problems of population and poverty in underdeveloped countries. These interests have been stimulated by the experience of teaching many students from such countries and by a commission I was given by the government of Mauritius. I was asked to advise that government on the provisions to be made for social security, health and welfare, bearing in mind the resources of Mauritius and the needs of its people.

At a first glance, this might seem a narrow and unexciting assignment. But as my two colleagues (Brian Abel-Smith and T.A. Lynes) and I became absorbed in the task, we came to see that we could not understand the problems unless they were set in a wider and deeper context (Titmuss et al, 1961). Analytically, we needed the spectacles of the historian, the anthropologist, the doctor, the political scientist and the economist. We were faced with a classical Malthusian situation made more complex by the impact of medical science; with a multiracial society composed of Hindus, Moslems, Chinese, French, British and Creoles; with a one-crop economy; with a declining national income per head; and with a confusion of cultures and religions exposed to many processes of cultures and religions exposed to many processes of change in structure, organisation and function.

As a microcosm of the problems of the underdeveloped world, Mauritius could be regarded, cynically or otherwise, as an absorbing social laboratory. Although small, and not as yet a battlefield for the conflicting ideologies of the West and the East, it presents many of the characteristics of the poorer, underdeveloped half of the world's population, particularly in Africa.

$$* * * * *$$

Mauritius, an island in the Indian Ocean about 500 miles east of Madagascar, is about a tenth of the size of Wales. In it is crammed a multiracial society of over 650,000 people – nearly half of them not yet 15 years old. About two thirds of these people are of Indian origin, with the Hindus outnumbering the Moslems as a political force by about three to one; 28% are of mixed African or Indian and European descent, known locally as 'Creole'; 3% are of Chinese origin and descent; and the remaining 2% are European, mostly of French origin. About a third of the population are Roman Catholics.

The Dutch, the French and the British have all in turn governed

Mauritius. Known as 'the Island of the Swan', it was ceded to Britain by the Treaty of Paris in 1814. The French brought in slaves from Africa to work the sugar plantations; the British brought in indentured labour from India later in the 19th century.

Since 1947, Mauritius has been moving rapidly towards some form of political independence. It now has universal suffrage and an Executive Council, most of whose members are elected. But there is little sense of social cohesion and complete political independence is both demanded and feared. The balance of views inevitably varies by ethnic group, income, class and religion. The mass of the people – Hindu, Moslem and Creole – are in transition from a primitive cash economy with strong and extensive kinship ties to a more Westernised way of life. Manual work is increasingly despised and resented. Everywhere there is a passion for education, but mostly for young men. English academic education has certainly left its imprint, but nothing remotely resembling an indigenous culture exists. Folk medicine, street hawkers of cheap penicillin imported from France, chains of rickety cinemas, and the more gaudy products of Hong Kong and Birmingham flourish side by side – in one of the loveliest islands of the world. The main centre for technical training in industrial crafts and skills is the central prison, architecturally modelled on Wormwood Scrubs. The rest of the population, if they aspire to educational advancement, learn about the kings and queens of England.

Economically speaking, sugar is the ruler of Mauritius. About 99% of al exports are sugar or sugar by-products, and the island relies on imports for nearly all its foodstuffs, clothing, other consumption goods, machinery and raw materials. The great sugar estates are chiefly in the hands of a few Franco-Mauritian families, nursed in the French culture, Catholic by religion, participating little in the life of the island and virtually unaware of the French Revolution. Although they run the estates with impressive technical efficiency, their attitude to the Indian labourers can only be described as old-fashioned.

* * * * *

Until 1947, it could hardly be said that Mauritius had a population problem. Then the World Health Organisation and teams of scientists from Britain intervened to control malaria. Since then, the rate of growth has been phenomenal – well over 3% per year, and one of the highest (if not the highest) in the world. It took Britain nearly 50 years to halve her infant mortality rate. Mauritius has done it in less than five years. Mass unemployment among young people is only one of the many consequences of the demographic changes brought about by medical science.

Rapidly declining mortality rates, combined with early marriage, unrestricted childbearing, the low status of women, strongly held religious beliefs, an economic system by which a large proportion of the population subsist on irregular and unpredictable cash earnings, a fatalistic attitude to life nurtured by custom, protein anæmia, and a long history of hardship, all point to an alarming future rise in numbers. My colleagues and I estimated that, if present trends continue, Mauritius will have a population of nearly three million by the end of the century – or a density of 4,000 people per square mile.

The effects of this rate of growth are already being felt. Despite a more efficient and relatively prosperous sugar industry and stable sugar prices during the 1950s, malaria control and other health measures have led to a decline in the national income per head of population and to a growth in unemployment. At a time when political control is passing from the British to the masses, these trends make it harder to create the conditions for an economic take-off through the development of local industry, food production and capital investment. Many arguments thus seem, on the surface, to point away from the introduction and expansion of what we in the West call 'social services': that is, the allocation of more resources for the provision of health, education and social security systems.

Population control, in the form of family limitation, is essential for economic growth. In the time available, it is the only non-violent answer to the threat of population disaster, but the encouragement of family limitation and the provision of facilities for the control of births cannot be considered in the abstract. Such measures, if they are to be effective in time, will depend on the systems of medical care and social welfare. What then are the priorities in the balance of economic and social development which are likely to help to slow down population expansion?

Advocates of family limitation often assume or imply that propaganda is the only, or main, instrument of change. Malthus believed in it passionately, but he was not faced with the difficulties of communal conflict in a multiracial society. He did, however, see that education, to be successful, needed a favourable social environment. He therefore wished to remove the counter-incentives for the procreation of large families. Hence his objection to the Poor Law, through which relief was often given according to the size of the family. In Mauritius, as in other African countries, the simple and negative approach of education and propaganda for family limitation cannot be adopted without similarly considering those elements in the cultural and social situation which are conducive to population growth.

In theory and in law, there is not (and never has been) any financial aid from public assistance in Mauritius for the unemployed and those with low and irregular cash earnings. But, while there is no overt relief for the unemployed and their families, those who are sick and are certified to be sick are eligible for assistance from the public system. This assistance embodies a highly complex formula – highly susceptible to abuse, if not administered by a classics don – which attempts to combine a number of mutually conflicting incentives for the kinship, as well as the sick individual. Whatever the theory, however, in practice it operates to encourage both large families and official sickness. Poverty in the demographic context of Mauritius is almost wholly a problem of poverty among children. The larger the family, the larger is the cash relief given to workers who are certified to be sick or 'fit for light work'. This Western euphemism, along with the incentives to be classified as sick, inevitably encourages resort, in an empirical fashion, to folk medicine, herbal remedies, other people's shrines, antibiotics or instalment credit from chemist's shops and, in particular, the government medical service. One consequence is that Mauritius – like other areas in Africa and the East – is now spending a higher proportion of its national income on the products of the pharmaceutical industry than the UK.

This heavy consumption of drugs is in part attributable to the public-assistance system. A structure of values has been created which increasingly makes it important to be regarded as sick; gives relief in cash or in kind, but generally refuses to provide modern drugs and injections; and thus leads the individual to the moneylender, the private doctor and the chemist's shop to buy drugs privately. These practices reinforce each other and, during the last 10 years of falling mortality, have been accompanied by a tenfold rise in the cost of public assistance.

This increasingly heavy burden on the island's budget is, however, due to unemployment rather than to a genuine rise in morbidity. A rapidly growing problem of unemployment is masquerading as sickness which is being partially relieved under public and charitable Poor-Law systems. Those who have large families are better off than those with small families. This system, modelled on the English Poor-Law system, encourages rather than discourages additions to already large families.

At the other end of the social scale, there is another system, also modelled on English law, which functions in a similar way. Child allowances in income tax are not only more generous as bonuses for large families than in the UK, but also include provision for private education overseas.

While it is paradoxical that two such powerful systems should exist in Mauritius with its menacing rates of population growth, it is necessary to remember that they were developed when the population was more or less stable. In the political and social circumstances of today [1962], neither could be abolished without substituting constructive alternative arrangements. All our proposals, and especially those for the reform of public assistance, were designed to discourage large families, early and rapid childbearing, and early marriage. In proposing deliberate and positive incentives in the reverse direction, we linked them closely with the provision and use of family-planning facilities.

$$* * * * *$$

Facilities for family planning cannot be provided on any scale in Mauritius – or in many other countries – outside the organised system of medical care. To be effective, provision has to be linked to applied Western medicine and its auxiliary or paramedical workers – nurses, midwives, dispensers, medical aids and pharmacists. If and when oral contraceptives become available at an economic price for the mass of the people, the same principle will hold; they will have to be provided under medical auspices (Lafitte, 1961).

But Mauritius is desperately short of doctors – a situation which prevails over virtually the whole of Africa. In common with other countries, Mauritius expends large sums of money annually to send overseas many of the brightest products of its slender secondary-school system to be trained in Western medicine. However, a substantial proportion do not return. Nor are the resources that are available always put to the best use. Because of the system of sickness relief, doctors in the government medical service in Mauritius spend much of their time, in effect, as public-assistance officers. In a population which has a high incidence of hookworm, tuberculosis and intestinal diseases, and in which perhaps half of the adults have tropical anæmias associated with protein deprivation, it is, moreover, a matter of great diagnostic difficulty to say that a worker is not fit when they present themselves with a variety of complaints. The search for doctors who will sign certificates and attempts to buy such certificates represent one of the subtler forms of what we in the West refer to as corrupting influences on professional conduct. Field (1957), examining the Russian medical scene, saw certification as the most important strategic role of the doctor in the social system. Because of its importance, the Soviet rulers reduced the medical profession to a docile, inert and poorly paid employee group.

In Mauritius, the existing system of poor relief, and the burden of certification, besides turning the doctor into a part-time unemployment clerk, have the further effect of making private practice more attractive, professionally and financially. As a result, private practice flourishes and large fortunes are being amassed in Mauritius as in many countries of tropical Africa today. The revolutionary impact of science on medicine over 20 years, in the form of drug therapy and other developments, is exerting a profound influence on the practice of medicine in Africa, partly because this eruption of science has preceded the growth of professional associations and ethical rules of conduct. In Britain and other Western countries, the doctor's role in society had evolved before the advent of the scientific age in medicine. In Mauritius and other low-income countries, however, there has not been time for the development of social controls and value systems. Outside the hospital, doctors work in professional isolation. They do not, therefore, develop a professional self-image, a definition of their role and a scale of values which, in the West, have been institutionalised in the form of a service motive and which are buttressed by many sanctions both within and without the profession. What the doctors learn as a value system in their training (which may be somewhat tenuous in the highly specialised medical curriculum of today) receives no further support when they return to their own country and set up in private practice.

In Mauritius, about a third of all the private doctors have holdings in chemists' shops. Branded products are prescribed which can be bought only at pharmacies in which the doctor has an interest. Streptomycin and other drugs which must be taken regularly for the effective control of tuberculosis are dispensed on a kind of pawnbroking system. The mishandling and misuse of these drugs in Mauritius (as in India and many African countries) means that drug-resistant tubercle bacilli are produced and disseminated to an alarming extent. The passion for injections at the site of the pain, which harmonises with the traditional practices of folk-doctors, is another reason for the prosperity of private practice and the unpopularity of government medicine. Newly qualified doctors are offered surgeries and financial aid by the pharmaceutical industry, which finds, among the eclectic and disease-ridden population of Mauritius, a ready market for its products.

These problems, which have to be identified if they are eventually to be resolved, are not peculiar to Mauritius. Gear (1960) has discussed the need for strong professional associations, with a backbone of independent doctors, in the newer African states and regretted that they seem unlikely to develop. "Medicine's true teachers and disciples", as he points out, "give more to Africa than medical care in a hospital or clinic". As it is, the rate of change in Africa has become almost unbearably rapid for both doctor and patient. It is almost as if penicillin and all the rest of these therapeutic weapons had been put into the hands of doctors in the West when they were secularised after the Renaissance.

* * * * *

Two general propositions emerge from this brief survey – with Mauritius as a case study – of the relation between the rate of scientific progress and the capacity of applied medicine to change. The first is that these scientific advances in the practice of medicine now need, for their efficacy, stricter professional codes of behaviour; that is, more explicit and comprehensive value systems of expected norms of medical behaviour derived from professional reference groups.

It is not, moreover, just a matter of efficacy – of whether the treatment works – but of doing harm to patients because of the potentially lethal instruments now wielded by modern medicine. This calls, among other things, for better communication between doctor and patient. Patients all over the world want two things from their doctor: science and humanity. In other words, technical competence and personal interest. Understandably, they are often confused and ambivalent about their preferences, for it is easier to recognise the latter than the former. This is because medicine, in becoming in part a science, has been transformed (like thermodynamics or nuclear physics) into something which can only be understood from within and after long study.

It follows – as a second proposition – that the greater the social and cultural differences between doctors practising Western medicine and their patients, the greater is the need for high standards of professional ethics. The fewer the differences in language, perception, behaviour, and modes of life, the easier understanding and treatment becomes, thus reducing the potential power of the doctor over the patient. These generalisations apply, of course, with added force in countries like Mauritius, where the cultural components of medical care are more important than in the West.

The situation in these countries has implications for Western countries in terms of recruitment, selection, training, deployment and professional organisation of doctors. For the UK, in particular, these are no longer purely domestic problems. Aid to the underdeveloped countries of the world is not solely a question of money and capital investment.

Part of the widening gap between the economically developed (or industrialised) and the less developed (or primary-producing) countries is caused by a faster rate of population growth. In the next 20 years, rates in most countries in Africa (including Mauritius) are likely to be more rapid than anywhere else in the world. But, if economic development is to take place, these rates must be checked. In Mauritius, this means that family-planning facilities must become an integral part of the system of medical care. The importance of social programmes for economic purposes must be recognised.

In the complex of social obstacles to economic growth in Mauritius, one of the most vital hinges will be medical science. To encourage the spread of family limitation, the Poor Law must be reformed; this depends in turn on the recruitment of more doctors and the development of professional ethics. And the answers to these questions are not to be found solely in Mauritius and other African states. They will have to be sought in the West.

Perhaps the one broad conclusion to be derived from this case study is that family planning, economic growth and social planning are indivisible. Medical science has helped to make them so; it has unwittingly assumed the responsibility of translating scientific progress into ethical practice.

Health and the welfare state

One point of view which is strongly held in the West (particularly the far West) is that welfare inhibits economic growth; it discourages thrift and savings; it encourages high absenteeism from work and low productivity; it diminishes family responsibility. An opposing point of view – equally strongly held – believes that welfare has more to do with humanitarian values than economic efficiency; with the social and ethical texture of society; with the exercise of compassion and reason in social relations.

Both these points of view have one thing in common. They are largely assertions and do not rest on any firm basis of fact. The concept of welfare has indeed suffered much in the past from stereotypes of deserving or undeserving recipients of charity; from images of well-meaning but muddle-headed social workers, cheerfully ignoring the harsh realities of economic life. We all drag about with us the chains of history – including an outdated one about the social worker – but it is time we recognised the evidence for a third point of view. Briefly, this is to see economic growth and social growth as interdependent in the sense that lagging behind in one has, necessarily, negative consequences on the other. Unbalanced economic growth may, for instance, generate a need for greater public expenditure than would otherwise be the case. The social costs of technological change, if allowed to lie where they fall, may result in larger costs in the future in the shape of physical and psychological problems, poverty, deprived children, ill-educated workers unable or unwilling to acquire new skills, and a general slackening in the sense of social involvement and participation in the life of community.

The case for social growth, in making a positive contribution to productivity as well as in reinforcing the social ethic of human equality, depends to a large extent on which forms of welfare are developed, how they are administered, and the education and skills of those who staff these services. We know now from experience in Britain that we did not abolish the spirit of the old and hated Poor Law by enacting new legislation in 1948. The same people – the same administrators and workers – still had to run the hospitals, public assistance offices and welfare services. They poured into the new social service bottles the old wine of discrimination and prejudice. What was needed was a major effort of training, retraining and separation of functions of administrators, social workers and local officials. This, I believe, is one of the less dramatic but important goals of welfare: a more humane and informed administration of social service. This is a prerequisite to 'reaching the unreachables' in our society. We have to realise that in this matter there is an enormous gap between the best we are capable of and what goes on; that reducing this gap is not simply an affair of spending more money; and that it is in great part the responsibility of public authorities to challenge whatever attitudes and conventions stand in the way of improvement, and to initiate the move to higher standards of service everywhere.

This is one of the major goals in the development of welfare as an aid to economic growth. It means efficient and more effective welfare. Before, however, turning to my next point, I must say something about the definition of the term. How do we define welfare? What are the main areas of collective action which may be designated as social policy?

I do not wish at this stage to embark on a long essay on definition. It will be sufficient to indicate the main areas of public (or publicly subsidised) social and welfare services, mainly:

1. education from the primary school to the university
2. medical care (preventive and curative)
3. housing and rent policies
4. income maintenance (including children's allowances, old age pensions, public assistance, and schemes for unemployment, sickness and industrial injuries benefits)
5. special services in kind for dependent groups, older people, deprived children, unsupported parents and various other groups with special needs

All these services are redistributive in their effects. They cannot be neutral, whether they are provided only for certain groups in the population or on the principle of universality. They change patterns of getting, spending and storing. In terms of total government expenditure, they may absorb anything from 10% to 30% of the annual budget.

In looking to the future and asking questions about the major objectives of these services, we must first inquire how they are functioning at present [1964] in the modern state. Are they in reality achieving what they were intended to achieve? To what extent and in what sectors are they redistributing resources on criteria of need or on criteria of productivity – on Myrdal's (1944) principle of cumulative causation? In attempting to answer such questions, we must also take account of the operations of the income tax system with all its complex indirect subsidies and transfers towards meeting the cost of different types of services and needs: for example, allowances for children, deductions for education, medical care, old age pensions, life assurance, owner-occupied houses and so forth. For those who pay income tax, these are welfare contributions and their general tendency in Britain and other countries is to reduce the progressiveness of the taxation system. They are, in short, redistributive in effect just as the formal welfare services are.

I cannot, of course, try to answer these important questions so far as other countries are concerned. However, from social policy studies in Britain and the US, it has become increasingly clear that certain tendencies are at work which conflict with the general model of a 'welfare state' redistributing resources in favour of the poor and those with the greatest need.

In Britain, for example, we have begun to ask statistical and sociological questions about the utilisation of the high-cost sectors of social welfare and the low-cost sectors of social welfare. We have been led to do so by the recognition that the Beveridge principle of universality in welfare – comprehensive systems of education, medical care and pensions for all citizens – does not, by itself alone, solve the problems of the underclass in our societies: that is, the fifth or quarter or more of the population who are badly educated, badly housed, badly fed and who often have greater need for medical care and services of many kinds than the general population.

Universality in welfare is needed – and was needed in Britain – to reduce and remove barriers of social and economic discrimination. Separate services for second-class citizens invariably become second-class services – whether they are organised for 10% or 50% of the population. Moreover, those who staff these services may come to believe that they themselves are second-class workers. Hence, when exercising discretionary powers in giving or withholding benefits and services, they may adopt a more punishing attitude to those of whom they may disapprove.

The principle of universality applied in 1948 to the main social welfare services in Britain was needed as a major objective favouring social integration; as a method of breaking down distinctions and discriminative tests between first-class and second-class citizens. But equal opportunity of access by right of citizenship to education, medical care and social insurance is not the same thing as equality of outcome. It is only a prerequisite – although a necessary one – to the objective of equalising the outcome. Other and more precise instruments of social policy are required in addition to achieve equality of outcome irrespective of race, religion or class.

I will now give a few examples of what we have been learning in the past 10 years [early 1950s to early 1960s] about the actual functioning of universally provided services in Britain.

1. Under the NHS, we have learnt that the higher income groups make better use of the NHS; they tend to receive more specialist attention; occupy more of the beds in better equipped hospitals; receive more elective surgery; have better maternity care; and are more likely to get psychiatric help and psychotherapy than

members of the so-called working classes – particularly the unskilled.

2. In the field of financial provision for old age (which dominated the budget for national insurance), we have learnt that the state now makes a larger contribution on average to the pensions of the rich than it does to the pensions of the poor. This has come about as a consequence of the combined action of the principle of universality, of tax allowances, subsidised pension schemes sponsored by employers, deductible life assurance and other factors.

3. Under the universal system of family allowances and children's allowances, a man earning £20,000 a year with two children will receive from the state (pay less tax) £5 a week for the children. At the other end of the scale, a man with two children and earning £500 a year will receive from the state 8/- a week. The rich father thus gets 13 times more from the state than the poor man in recognition of the dependent needs of children.

4. In the field of housing, the subsidy paid by the state to owner-occupiers of many categories of houses is on average greater than the subsidy received by most tenants of public housing (local government) schemes. This has come about as a consequence of the differential effects of local rate payments, housing subsidies, interest rates, tax deductibles for mortgage interest, and other factors. To arrive at this conclusion for housing (as for pensions and benefits for children) calls for a complex and intensive analysis of many diverse systems of government intervention.

5. For my last example, I take education. Next to the ownership of land and property, this (and the lack of it) is today the most revolutionary and explosive force in developed and developing economies. Earning power, life chances, achievement, position and class, and even the level of pension in old age depend on education and training, and on society's investment of scarce resources in those who are educated. In highly developed countries, the total value of the capital sunk in the education of the population is immense. It has been estimated for the US that in 1957 the capital sunk in the education of the population represented 40% of the total of physical tangible capital plus intangible educational capital (Schultz, 1963, p 51).

This, of course, is not to say that education can be viewed simply as another form of productive capital investment. It confers other benefits: social and spiritual. It enables the educated person to enjoy more freedom and a fuller life. But education does have value as a straightforward commercial investment. The return on higher education as a purely commercial investment for the individual is probably larger today in most Western countries than any other form of investment. If heavily financed by the state, and if proportionately more children from better-off homes benefit, then the system will be redistributive in favour of the rich.

In the past, the spread of the first stages of education to all children – the principle of universality – was a major equalising and integrating force in our societies We are now entering in the West a new era in which secondary and higher education may become one of the major disequalising and socially disruptive forces. There are three reasons for this.

One is that scarce resources only allow a small proportion of young people access to good secondary and higher education. (The principle of universality cannot be applied to higher education in any country of the world in the 20th century.)

The second reason is a greatly intensified problem of earnings and labour forgone (associated, of course, with the problem of educational motivation) which leads to the exclusion of working-class children. Immense sacrifices are called for from parents and children living in poor conditions and bad housing, if earnings are given up in favour of study.

And the third reason, is that, as industrial, scientific and technological developments demand more people with higher education, there will be, as in Britain, pressures to invest more scarce resources in such education at the expense of education for the masses, and also to concentrate secondary education on those who will go on to higher education. These pressures, we must recognise, are growing stronger in our societies.

These five examples I have given of trends and tendencies in the functioning of social welfare services provide us with some glimpses of the magnitude of the task that lies ahead in redefining the goals of welfare. The major beneficiaries of the high-cost sectors of social welfare are the middle- and upper-income classes. The poor make more use of certain services (for instance, public assistance) but these tend on a per capita basis to be the low-cost sectors.

In addition to these trends, Britain and other Western countries have experienced in the last 15 years a rapid growth in what we may call 'non-wage income'. This has taken the form of services, fringe benefits, privileges and prerequisites which are not generally or wholly subject to tax. The major beneficiaries have been the middle- and upper-income groups.

In short, we can now say that the advent of 'the welfare state' in Britain after the Second World War has not led to any significant redistribution of income and wealth in favour of the poorer classes. According to the most recent estimates (Revell, 1964, p 27), 5% of the population of the UK owned 87% of all personal wealth in 1911–13, 79% in 1936-38 and 75% in 1960. The decline in the concentration of wealth, although insignificant over the period of 50 years, is less marked since 1938 than during the years of mass unemployment and economic depression between 1913 and 1938. The trend towards a somewhat less unequal concentration in the ownership of wealth appears to have slowed down in the past 25 years [up to 1963]. This is all the more remarkable when we consider the effects from 1938 of substantially higher rates of taxation and estate duty, the equalising forces of the Second World War, full employment and a far greater employment of married women, and the supposedly redistributive effects of 'the welfare state'. Full employment for nearly 20 years, considered alone, might have been expected to have brought about a markedly less unequal concentration; a much greater proportion of workers have had opportunities of accumulating some savings.

Moreover, it has to be remembered that all these figures are expressed in terms of *individual* holdings. We do know from various studies that, since the 1930s, there has been an increasing tendency for large owners of property to distribute their wealth among their families (Titmuss, 1962b, Chapter 5). The British fiscal system is almost unique in the Western world in its generous treatment of wealth-holders in allowing them to use family settlements, discretionary trusts, gifts, family covenants and other legal devices for redistributing and rearranging income and wealth. This trend is reflected in the startling fact that, in the mid-1950s and within age groups, it was in the young adult age group that the tendency for wealth to be concentrated in a few hands was most marked. If it were possible to measure the distribution of wealth in terms of family holdings, it might thus be found that inequality had increased since 1938. There is certainly evidence from the US, which has experienced a marked increase in individual wealth inequality since 1949, that measurement in terms of family holdings does make a significant difference (Lampman, 1959).

Yet, since the end of the 1930s, it has been the broad intention of welfare measures to facilitate a more equal distribution of economic resources. Why then, it may be asked, have these unintended consequences of social policy come about? For one thing, our conceptual frame of reference was too narrow and too romantic. We have associated 'welfare' with the 'poor'; it has given us a nice feeling. Second, we too readily assumed that social legislation solves social problems. As every social worker knows (or should know), it does not. Third, we failed to develop in the 1950s techniques of social analysis as we have developed techniques of economic analysis. Fourth, we have tended to compartmentalise welfare; to put it in a separate conceptual box; to see it as a hindrance to economic growth in the long run – as it may be in the short run. Accordingly, therefore, we failed to relate the functioning of services and the measurement of social need with the dynamics of change – economic, technological, social and psychological.

Lastly, we lacked vision and social inventiveness. We did not see that the task of reaching the poor and minority groups, of redistributing resources in their favour, of getting them to use and benefit from health, education and social services, was a far more formidable one than most reformers imagined. We gravely under-estimated the growing strength of the forces working in the other direction – forces stemming from economic and technological change, specialisation and the class division of society. And we failed to grasp the importance of the connections between, for instance, bad housing and the inability to profit from education; between an inadequate command over language and the need for more social workers to help to interpret and manipulate the resources of a complex society; and between social policies and the inadequacy of the administrative machine (particularly at local levels) to translate policies into effective action.

In short, because we were complacent, because we looked inwards and backwards to the 1930s, our social diagnosis was inadequate. Only now are we coming to see that we need much sharper tools of social study and measurement; more precise social analyses of conditions, needs and the actual functioning of services; more attempts at social planning in alliance with economic planning. How many hospital beds shall we need in 1975? How many more social workers, welfare workers and other staff will be required? What problems of crime, delinquency and deprivation will confront our societies in 10 years' time?

These and similar questions are admittedly difficult ones to answer, but, if we wish to redefine the goals of welfare, then we cannot escape the responsibility of being more intelligent about what is happening and what is likely to happen in our societies.

We shall not make progress in identifying and measuring the future tasks of welfare unless we relate need and response to the ongoing forces of change. If we accept that two of the major positive goals of welfare are (i) to increase and spread the impact of equalising factors, and (ii) to speed up the impact of factors favouring integration, then we must base the many practical details of policy and action on a more informed diagnosis of change. From recent advances in the social sciences, we can be reasonably sure about the continuation of certain trends, for example.

To achieve economic growth and innovation, modern societies need to apply the lessons of advances in technology and science. This means more division of labour and specialisation; more education and specialised training; more specificity in manpower recruitment and deployment; longer hierarchies in occupational positions in the labour force; larger incentives for training and mobility; more and probably larger differentials in rewards. These processes, necessary as they are, tend on balance to generate disequalising forces and, by demanding higher standards of education, training and acquired skills, they can make more difficult the task of integrating people with different cultural backgrounds and levels of motivation. While we may raise expectations in people's minds about what the future may hold, technology simultaneously raises the barriers to entry. This process is believed to be partly responsible for the solidifying of a permanent underclass of deprived citizens, uneducated, unattached and alternating between apathetic resignation and frustrated violence.

A second process, built-in among modern societies and related to technological change, is represented by the growth of professionalism. In Britain and other countries, the professions are largely recruited from the middle classes; professional workers come from homes and educational institutions where they have little contact with manual workers and people from different cultures. Thus, they bring to their work middle-class values in the processes of giving or withholding medical care, education, legal aid and welfare benefits. Their model of the ideal pupil, student, patient and client is one with middle-class values and a middle-class tongue (Bernstein, 1964). This process, subtle and often unconscious, partly explains why in Britain, under universally available welfare services, the middle classes tend to receive better services and more opportunities for advancement. This is understandable: we all prefer the cooperative patient or client, motivated to achievement, anxious to learn, anxious to work. Of all professions in contact with the poor, only social workers in their training learn to understand the significance of this factor in their relationships. They recognise the importance of guarding professionalism against functioning as a disequalising force.

While I have not attempted any precise description of today's welfare goals, I believe that some of them are implicit in the lessons of experience. These I have set within the context of certain general principles of economic management. In doing so, I have stated a case for a balance of economic and social growth. We want higher productivity for a higher standard of living and we want a more equal society. We want individual advancement and we want an integrated community of self-respecting human beings. In achieving these goals, systems of welfare have a major contribution to make. They will, of course, present us time and time again with conflicting ideologies and conflicting policies.

In the choices that we have to make I would like, in conclusion, as a student of welfare, to offer two personal prescriptions.

The world desperately needs standard-bearers of social inventiveness and personal integrity; examples to look up to; precepts to learn from. In a world made smaller by modern communications, what we do in the field of welfare and how we do it has an influence far outside national boundaries. People are still moved by the ideas of compassion. So we need pioneers in the art of giving. Second, I believe that, when conflict in policies presents itself, we should take risks in welfare choices. We should trust rather than distrust people and put our faith in the ultimate reasonableness of human beings.

To me, the 'welfare state' has no meaning unless it is positively and constructively concerned with redistributive justice and social participation. These goals may collide in the short run with the need to increase economic productivity and to raise the general standard of living. Although we cannot be sure that this collision is inevitable, it is, nevertheless, tempting to argue – tempting to take the safe side – that, when we are richer, we can afford to be more generous to the less fortunate. But, equally, can we be sure that, in the processes of getting richer and of concentrating only on getting richer, we shall not, as a society, lose the impetus to create a more equal and socially just community?

Epilogue:
Richard Titmuss's contribution to the sociology of health and illness

Raymond Illsley

The published work of Richard Titmuss stretches over 35 years of deep and sometimes turbulent change. His research was motivated by a powerful urge to improve the health and the social life of his fellow citizens, particularly the poor. It therefore reflected the live issues of contemporary social and political events. The creation of the National Health Service in 1948 marked a sharp dividing line in his work on health. In the earlier period, Titmuss addressed social injustice and its impact on death and health; in the later period, he dealt with the issues involved in managing the newly achieved NHS and the emerging welfare state. They are the phases of the health debate described by Klein (2001) as the politics of creation and the politics of consolidation. The linking theme for Titmuss was always the search for social equality.

* * * * *

Some of the earlier issues that he felt he had to address (Titmuss, 1938, 1943) illustrate the enormous shift in public thought occurring during his writing years. Do the high birth rates of the poor inevitably lead to a fall in the national stock of intelligence? Does the lowering of the infant death rate, particularly in the poorer classes, produce a nation of the unfit? Even now, every decade seems to produce some eminent proponent of such theories, but they were persistent widely held concerns when Titmuss wrote his early books. Possible falls in national health and intelligence resulting from low middle-class birth rates were a strong factor in setting up the Royal Commission on Population. Scotland went so far as to conduct a massive survey of child IQ as a first step in testing the theory. Its most extreme form, quoted by Titmuss (1938), came from the then President of the Royal College of Physicians, "One cannot help wondering, indeed, whether the stinting production and the careful saving of infant lives to-day is really, biologically speaking, as wholesome as the mass production and lavish scrapping of the last century".

I first became aware of Titmuss in 1951 when, as a social scientist,

I joined a multi-disciplinary team studying the social and biological causes of stillbirth and first-week death in Aberdeen. It emerged that, during the war years, the team leader, Dugald Baird, on periodic visits to London to attend meetings of the Royal Commission on Population, had called on Titmuss at the War Department where he was collecting material for the official history of the war. They sketched out ideas for a post-war research project, attractive to Baird as an unusually social-minded obstetrician and to Titmuss as a radical social analyst. When Titmuss joined Jerry Morris at the newly established Medical Research Council Social Medicine Research Unit in 1948, they helped Baird to put these ideas into practice.

Sociology was then a rare commodity in Britain and sociology applied to health barely existed. Titmuss's material consisted of decennial census statistics, the annual reports of medical officers of health reaching back into the 19th century, and the reports of a few inquiries by the Ministry of Health, Poor Law Commissioners, and so on. These were supplemented by the research findings of a few socially minded public health officers and, more rarely, clinicians. Titmuss was deeply aware of the lack of first-hand, research-based evidence, but was also aware that the existing sources had been inadequately exploited – startling findings hidden by dead-pan numerical description and perhaps unwillingness to draw attention to the state of the poor. He saw himself carrying out the recommendation of a contemporary epidemiologist: "... all this light on contemporary social conditions should not be imprisoned between the covers of a Blue-book, but should illumine our understandings and our hearts, teaching us to work for a better England".

I have found no single place where Titmuss systematically set out his ideas and conclusions in a theoretical form. However, a review across the pre-war and wartime books reveals the development of a remarkably comprehensive theory of the relationships between social structure and social change, on the one hand, and the determinants of physical and intellectual health and development, on the other. He saw that the unequal distribution of wealth caused a massive and unnecessary loss of life at all ages but particularly at six to twelve months of age, broadly declining across the following years but still substantial into late middle age. The big geographical differences between the industrial North and the more prosperous South East were clearly attributable to poverty, there being little difference between social class I rates in these extreme areas. The biggest class and regional differences occurred in relation to those diseases with a clear and accepted environmental base.

Constant falls across previous decades, as a result of increased levels of living, of public health measures and scientific progress, had made nonsense of the still fashionable concept of an 'irreducible minimum'. The well-to-do had been able to "avail themselves at a greater rate than the poor of the knowledge and opportunities for better infantile health which, in theory, are available to all". The relative gap between class death rates had not narrowed; indeed, for some age groups it had increased, the class V rate lagging behind its class I equivalent by 20 or 30 years. "The rigidity of the class structure holds, it seems, in the field of health just as it does in the realm of money... For the period we have covered, the social structure has become increasingly immobilized; yet all the time the illusion of social mobility has been gently fostered."

"From the moment of conception the minutiae and the majesty of money come into play." The health differential was greatest in the first year of life as the vulnerable infant became increasingly exposed to a frequently hostile environment. A high death rate meant a high damage rate in the survivors. These then became further exposed, and that experience continued to damage and to impair physical development across the school years and into adult life. Intellectual development was subject to the same interweaving of social and health experiences. Titmuss saw the 'social training' of the child in the pre-school years as a highly significant period in children's lives, inevitably affected by maternal health and knowledge: "If the beginning be sordid, can life be full, abundant and generous?".

While there are many passing references in Titmuss's early work to the inadequacy of medical care, the emphasis was on inequality, and specifically on poverty in its direct impact on health, and also poverty as an environment. Poverty did not just mean low or uncertain incomes; it was a short-hand expression for unemployment, overcrowding, shortage of food or warmth, unhygienic living conditions, inadequate clothing and, most inclusive of all, 'life without interest'. While it was possible to trace particular illnesses to the effect of specific elements of poverty, the overwhelming emphasis was on poverty/environment as the fundamental cause, implying that poverty is indivisible.

This is a powerful theory. Its principal theme was firmly based on demographic, sociological and epidemiological analysis, the outer edges being more intuitive and speculative in the absence of the detailed data of today's world. Available literature was pushed to its explanatory limits and fuzzy indicative words and phrases such as 'life without interest' did not lend themselves to scientific testing. Results from thousands of studies about inequalities in health have been published in the subsequent 60 years. They have added detail, especially by tracing the pathways through which social experience becomes translated into illness. They have made no serious dents in the major theoretical components of Titmuss's argument. Indeed, the emphasis he placed on childhood social experience and its continuing repercussions into adult life, socially, physically and intellectually, is only now being fully recognised (Acheson, 1998; Illsley, 2002).

In later years he reviewed what had been achieved. The nation's health had improved and it enjoyed a relative affluence. Both health and income differentials had not only persisted but widened. As the cruder injustices of the past were replaced by new and milder forms, he foresaw a danger that greater affluence would obscure the continued presence of inequality. He sensed a retreat of governments from responsibility for promoting equality. "The Beveridge principle of universality in welfare does not, by itself alone, solve the problems of the underclass in our society" (Titmuss, 1968a, p 91). Diagnosis and prognosis have proved accurate. We move from Titmuss through Black (1980) to Acheson (1998), from infant mortality through lung cancer and heart disease to lifestyle and the quality of life. With scientific medicine and ameliorative social policy, we tackle each of the health symptoms of inequality as they arise, but the driving force in Titmuss's theory – the inequalities inherent in our political, social and economic system, barely touched by policy – ensures persistence of the problem.

This, of course, was not the viewpoint in the late 1940s and the 1950s when Titmuss was writing about health and the NHS. He knew, we knew, that the health of the nation could not be created by medical services, but disbelief was suspended in the euphoria of massive social reform. Long-held visions were being implemented. Full employment and the new social security measures would get rid of poverty. The new National Health Service would give free access to medical treatment for everybody. The immediate task was to implement and, for a few such as Titmuss, to monitor.

The scale of the enterprise was daunting: "At a legislative stroke 1,000 hospitals owned and run by a variety of voluntary bodies and 540 hospitals owned by the local authorities were nationalized. At the same time free practitioner care, hitherto limited to 21 million people covered by the insurance scheme set up by Lloyd George in 1911, was extended to the entire population" (Klein, 2001, p 1). These and all supporting services and staff had to be welded into a single organisation. The structures and guiding procedures for each organisational component were the result, not of prior experience – it was a unique form of service – nor of applying technical, organisational expertise – such knowledge barely existed – but of bargaining between political, administrative and professional participants.

Over the 1950s and 1960s, Titmuss wrote what now appears as a running commentary on the key issues confronting the NHS. Some questions recur frequently. Can general practice be transformed from its degraded pre-war status and function to take a new responsibility as a scientifically informed and efficient social service? What would be the relationship between the new general practice and the higher status consultants in their hospital setting? To whom should the doctor be accountable in society? How could tendencies to both scientific and bureaucratic complexity be controlled and how could the self-perceived needs of patients be recognised and met? These are all issues that have constantly recurred across the history of the NHS to the present day. The only major troublesome issue persisting through into the new millennium to which Titmuss gave little attention is the role of government in the control of the medical profession and of NHS health priorities. This reflects the fact that, for much of the 1950s, the NHS was not the subject of political debate and that a concordat about the respective roles of state and the medical profession had been forged in the negotiations leading up to its foundation.

It would be easy to pick out from Titmuss's commentaries on the NHS a variety of specific themes and to say: this is how he contributed to the sociology of science, of the professions, of organisations, or of health and illness. However, to do so would be to miss his characteristic approach. He did indeed deal with these concepts, but he dealt with them in combination. He showed an abiding interest in scientific progress and its impact on the reduction of pain or the saving of life. But he was careful to stress that this influence, seen by many as the key factor in post-war achievements in health, was only one of many contributory influences. The efficient and effective use of new drugs or surgical techniques depended on the system whereby resources were distributed and the medical professions organised to make the best use of them. Both factors, science and organisation, were individually important, but they also acted on each other and affected the thought, behaviour and status of all the major participants in health care: GPs, consultants and patients.

In his pre-NHS studies of differential death and his work on the wartime emergency health service, Titmuss (1950) had seen the chaotic and degraded state of general practice. The single-handed GP whose "specialism lay in his own personality, armed with little besides a stethoscope, a thermometer and a personal accumulation of bedside observations" (Titmuss, 1958, p 192), was in no position to make use of the new knowledge. The GP should, and could, be the link between patients and high technology, an informed social service. In one sense, the creation of the NHS had further degraded GPs by making some of their personal skills irrelevant, by excluding them from hospital work and simultaneously emphasising the scientific medical skills of the consultant. By 1963, however, Titmuss perceived a "beginning in the process of establishing a social framework in which the great majority of general practitioners ... may find a more assured and satisfying role than was their lot before 1948" (1968a, p 155). He saw this as a process of adjustment, partly to the challenge of scientific medicine, but also to the "rising standards of expectations of medical care from a more articulate, health–conscious society" (1958, p 155). That adjustment has indeed taken place but it took 40 tense years of protest, crisis, negotiation and reorganisation to transform the position and power of general practice into the primary care social service that Titmuss envisaged.

Nor was specialised medicine in its hospital setting in a position to take advantage of the vast developments in science and bring them out of the laboratory into the practice of medicine. This required reorganisation of hospitals away from the chaos, diversity and frequent penury of the voluntary/local authority system. Titmuss acknowledged the 'inestimable gains' achieved by scientific medicine in the NHS, but he had reservations. With increasing complexity, the growth of professional syndicalism and the fragmentation of disciplines, and the need for precision and accuracy in applied sciences, there were dangers for the system and for the patient. In the preoccupation with means, the sight of the goals might be obscured. It would be more difficult than in simpler organisations to treat the patient as a person. In a complex and changing institution, there was also the danger that such deficiencies might not be identified or that they would be ignored. On these, as so many other topics, he called for more data, more transparency, more externally originated research – more Florence Nightingales.

Concern for the patient, the third participant in these interactions, is frequently voiced, but the patient is a more shadowy figure than the GP or the consultant. Much had been written about the medical professions and their views had often been expressed in the period leading up to the NHS. People as patients had received little attention; the government and political parties were seen as proxies for the individual consumer. The wealth of material from sociological studies about health beliefs and behaviour was not yet available. Titmuss saw the patient as vulnerable in the face of the new scientific medicine. He was concerned about the dehumanising of the individual into a 'case' and the impact of tendencies to authoritarian attitudes. On the other hand, he saw the future patient as more informed, more aware of the meaning of health to life and career, and more articulate. Recent studies had already shown the middle classes as more conscious of the need for health in their lives and more aware of the technical potentialities of modern medicine. They made better use of the NHS, got more specialist attention, more elective surgery, and more psychiatric help and psychotherapy. That conclusion remains relevant.

The ideas that I have described were not based on empirical studies; they had not been tested by research. They derived from personal observations and a scarce literature. The social scientists, later regarded as the forerunners of medical sociology (although they had trained in other disciplines), were so few as late as 1958 that they held their informal meetings in small hotels with only five bedrooms so that they could take over the residents' lounge for their discussions. Titmuss provided organised ideas for them and their successors to test and elaborate. It is remarkable how many of those ideas have proved relevant to the history of health and health policy over the subsequent 30 years.

General bibliography

Abel-Smith, B. (1964) *The hospitals, 1800-1948: A study in social administration in England and Wales*, London: Heinemann.

Abel-Smith, B. and Titmuss, R.M. (1956) *The cost of the National Health Service in England and Wales*, Cambridge: Cambridge University Press.

Abel-Smith, B. and Townsend, P. (1965) *The poor and the poorest*, Occasional Papers on Social Administration, no 17, London: G Bell and Sons.

Acheson, D. (1998) *Independent Inquiry into Inequalities in Health*, London: The Stationery Office.

Alcock, P., Glennerster, H., Oakley, A. and Sinfield, A. (eds) (2001) *Welfare and wellbeing: Richard Titmuss's contribution to social policy*, Bristol: The Policy Press.

Armstrong, D. (2002) 'The gaze', in C. Blakemore (ed) *The Oxford companion to the body*, Oxford: Oxford University Press.

Bach, F., Hill, N.G., Preston, T.W. and Thornton, C.E. (1939) *Annals of Rheumatic Diseases*, vol 1, p 210.

Barker, D.J.P. (1992) *Fetal and infant origins of adult disease*, London: BMJ Publishing.

Barker, D.J.P. (1998) *Mothers and babies and health in later life*, Edinburgh: Churchill Livingstone.

Barker, J. (1980) 'The relationship of informal care to formal social services: who helps people deal with social and health problems if they arise in old age?', in S. Lonsdale, A. Webb and T. Briggs (eds) *Teamwork in personal social services and health care*, London/New York, NY: Personal Social Services Council/Syracuse University Press.

Barker, J. (1985) 'Health promotion in later life: a community challenge', in F. Glendinning (ed) *New initiatives in self-health for older people*, London/Stoke on Trent: The Health Education Council/Beth Johnson Foundation.

Barker, J. (1993) 'Editorial: Ageing and later life', *International Journal of Epidemiology and Community Health*, vol 47, pp 81-3.

Bartley, M.J. (2004) *Health inequality*, Cambridge: Polity Press.

Bartley, M.J., Ferrie, J. and Montgomery, S.M. (1999) 'Living in a high-unemployment economy: understanding the health consequences', in M.G. Marmot and R.J. Wilkinson (eds) *Social determinants of health*, Oxford: Oxford University Press.

Bartley, M.J., Carpenter, L., Dunnell, K. and Fitzpatrick, R. (1995) 'Measuring inequalities in health: an analysis of mortality patterns using two social classifications', *Sociology of Health and Illness*, vol 18, no 4, pp 455-74.

Bell, D, (1961) *The end of ideology: On the exhaustion of political ideas in the fifties*, New York, NY: Collier Books.

Bengtson, V. and Schaie, K. (1995) *Handbook of theories of aging*, New York, NY: Springer.

Berkeley, C., Bonney, V. and MacLeod, D. (1938) *The abnormal in obstetrics*, London: E. Arnold & Co.

Bernstein, B. (1964) *British Journal of Sociology*, vol 15, no 1.

Black Report (1980) *Inequalities in health: Report of a research working group*, DHSS, London: HMSO [reissued in 1999 by The Policy Press].

Bloom, S. (1965) *The doctor and his patient: A sociological interpretation*, New York, NY: Macmillan.

Brady, D.S. (1965) *Age and the income distribution*, Research Report no 8, Social Security Administration, WA: US Department of Health.

Brewster, A.W. and Seldowitz, E. (1962) *Public Health Reports*, vol 77, no 9, Washington, WA: US Public Health Service.

British Medical Association (1905) *Report on Contract Practice, British Medical Journal Supplement*, 22 July.

British Medical Association (1909) *Secret remedies: What they cost and what they contain*, London: British Medical Association.

Brown, R. E. (1959), *Principles for planning the future hospital system*, no 721, Washington, WA: US Public Health Service.

Bunbury, H. and Titmuss, R.M. (1957) *Lloyd George's ambulance wagon (the memoirs of W.J. Braithwaite)*, London: Methuen.

Carter, R. (1958) *The doctor business* [publisher unknown].

Charles-Jones, H., Latimer, J. and May, C. (2003) 'Transforming general practice: the redistribution of medical work in primary care', *Sociology of Health and Illness*, vol 25, no 1, pp 71-92.

Chief Medical Officer (1940) *Health of the school child, 1938*, Annual report of the Chief Medical Officer of the Ministry of Education, London: HMSO.

Churchill, E. (1949) in N.W. Faxon (ed) *The hospital in contemporary life*, Cambridge, MA: Harvard University Press.

Clark-Kennedy, A.E. (1950) *The Lancet*, vol 2, p 661.

Clark-Kennedy, A.E. (1955) *British Medical Journal*, vol 1, p 619.

Close, H.G. (1930) *Guy's Hospital Report*, No 80, p 372.

Cloward, R.A. and Elman, R.M. (1966) 'Poverty, injustice and the welfare state', *Nation*, 28 February.

Coborn, A.F. (1931) *The factor of infection in the rheumatic state*, Baltimore, MD: Williams & Wilkins.

Cochrane, A. and Clarke J. (eds) (1993) *Comparing welfare states: Britain in international context*, London: Sage Publications and the Open University.

Coe, R. (1970) *Sociology of medicine*, New York, NY: McGraw-Hill.

Coombs, C.F. (1924) *Rheumatic heart disease*, Bristol: John Wright & Sons.

Cox, A. (1950) *British Medical Journal*, vol 1, p 78.

Crouch, C. (2003) *Commercialisation or citizenship: Education policy and the future of public services*, London: Fabian Society.

Curtis Committee (1946) *Report of the Care of Children Committee*, Cmd 6922, London: HMSO.

Dale, H.H. (1950) *British Medical Journal*, vol 1, p 1.

Davis, M.M. (1955) *Medical care for tomorrow*, New York, NY: Harper & Row.

Dean, H. (2004) 'Reconceptualising dependency, responsibility and rights', in H. Dean (ed) *The ethics of welfare: Human rights, dependency and responsibility*, Bristol: The Policy Press.

De Graff, A.C. and Ling, C. (1935) *American Heart Journal*, vol 10, p 459.

De Tocqueville, A. (1946) *Democracy in America* ('The World's Classics' edn), Oxford: Oxford University Press.

Dicey, A.V. (1905) *Lecture on the relation between law and opinion in England during the nineteenth century*, London: Macmillan & Co.

Dicey, A.V. (1926) *Lecture on the relation between law and opinion in England in the nineteenth century* (2nd edn), London: Macmillan & Co.

Dunnell, K. and Dix, D. (2000) 'Are we looking forward to a longer and healthier retirement?', *Health Statistics Quarterly*, vol 6, pp 18-25.

Durkheim, E. (1957) *Professional ethics and civic morals*, trans. C. Brookfield, London: Routledge & Kegan Paul.

Eckstein, H (1955), *Political Quarterly*, vol xxvi, no 4.

Economist, The (1944) 'Condition of the people', 30 December, pp 859-60.

Ellis, J.R. (1956) 'Changes in medical education', *The Lancet*, vol 1, p 813.

Elman, R. (1966) *The poorhouse state: The American way of life on public assistance*, New York, NY: Pantheon Books.

Estes, C., Biggs, S. and Phillipson, C. (2003) *Social theory, social policy and old age: A critical introduction*, Buckinghamshire: Open University Press.

Field, M. (1957) *Doctor and patient in Soviet Russia*, Cambridge, MA: Harvard University Press.

Fitts, W.T. and Fitts, B. (1955) 'Ethical standards of the medical profession', *The Annals of the American Academy of Political and Social Science*, January, p 21.

Fox, T.F. (1951) *The Lancet*, vol 2, p 173.

Freeman, H., Levine, S. and Reeder, L. (1973) *Handbook of medical sociology*, Princeton, NJ: Prentice-Hall.

Friedson, E. (1961, 1980) *Patients' views of medical practice*, New York, NY: Russell Sage Foundation.

Freidson, E. (1970) *Professional dominance: The social structure of medical care*, Chicago, Il: Aldine.

Friedman, M. (1962) *Capitalism and freedom*, Chicago, IL: University of Chicago Press.

Gardner, F. and Witts, L.J. (1946) 'Length of stay in hospital', *The Lancet*, vol 2, p 392.

Garrod, L.P (1955) *British Medical Journal*, vol 2, p 756.

Gear, H.S. (1960) 'Medicine in the New Africa', *The Lancet*, vol 2, p 1020.

General Register Office (1958, 1960, 1962) *Morbidity Statistics from General Practice*, London.

Giddens, A. (1974) *Positivism and sociology*, London: Heinemann.

Gillie Committee (1963) *The field of work of the family doctor*, Report of the Standing Medical Advisory Committee to the Central Health Services Council, London: HMSO.

Glass, D.V. (1954) *Social mobility*, London: Routledge.

Glendinning, C., Coleman, A. and Rummery, K. (2002) 'Partnerships, performance and primary care: developing integrated services for older people in England', *Ageing and Society*, vol 22, pp 185-208.

Glover, J.A. (1930) *The Lancet*, vol 1, pp 499 and 607.

Glover, J.A. (1934) *Proceedings of the Royal Society of Medicine*, vol 24, p 953.

Glover, J.A. (1943) *The Lancet*, vol 2, p 51.

Goffman, E. (1963) *Stigma: Notes on the management of spoiled identity*, Englewood Cliffs, NJ: Prentice-Hall.

Goodall, J.W.D. (1952) *The Lancet*, vol 1, p 807.

Gordon, R. (1999) 'Kant, Smith and Hegel: the market and the categorical imperative', in F. Trentmann (ed) *Paradoxes of civil society: New perspectives on modern German and British history*, Oxford: Berghahn.

Gramm, S. (1962) 'The small scale hospital and optional organization of community health procedures', *Conference Paper on the Economics of Health and Medical Care*, MI: University of Michigan.

Grant, R.T. (1933) *Heart*, vol 6, p 275.

Gray, P.G. and Cartwright, A. (1953) 'Government social survey', *The Lancet*, vol 2, p 1308.

Grundy, E. (2003) 'The epidemiology of ageing', in R. Tallis and H. Sillit (eds) *Brocklehurst's textbook of geriatric medicine and gerontology* (6th edn), London: Churchill Livingstone.

Grundy, F. (1944) *A note on the virtual statistics of Luton*, Luton [publisher unknown].

Grundy, F. and Titmuss, R.M. (1945) *Report on Luton*, Luton: The Seagrave Press.

Guillebaud Committee (1956) *Committee of Enquiry into the cost of the National Health Service*, London: HMSO.

Hadfield, S.J. (1953), *British Medical Journal*, vol 2, p 691.

Hall, A. (1956) *British Medical Journal*, vol 2, p 57.

Hamilton, J.A (1961) *Patterns of hospital ownership and control*, Minneapolis, MN: University of Minnesota Press.

Hardy, H. Nelson (1901) *The state of the medical profession in Great Britain and Ireland in 1900*, Dublin: Fannin & Co.

Hardy, J.D., Wolff, H.G. and Goodell, H. (1952) *Pain sensations and reactions*, in *Facsimile of 1952 edition* (1967), New York, NY: Hafner.

Hart, D'Arcy, P.M. and Wright, G.P. (1939) *Tuberculosis and social conditions*, London: National Association for the Prevention of Tuberculosis.

Hawley, P.B. (1952), 'Surgeons look at fee-splitting', *Hospitals*, September.

Hayes, J.H. (ed) (1954) *Factors affecting the cost of hospital care* [publisher unknown].

Hedley, O.F. (1936) *Public Health Bulletin, Washington*, pp 23 and 55.

Henrich, J. (2001) 'In search of homo economicus: behavioural experiments in 15 small-scale societies', *American Economic Review*, vol 91, pp 73–8.

Herbert, S.M. (1939) *Britain's health. Prepared by S. Mervyn Herbert on the basis of the Report on Britain's health services by Political and Economic Planning*, Harmondsworth: Penguin.

Hill, N.G. (1930) *British Journal of Childhood Diseases*, vol 27, p 161.

Illsley, R. and Kincaid, J.C. (1963) 'Social correlations of perinatal mortality', in N.R. Butler and D.G. Bonham (eds) *Perinatal mortality*, Edinburgh: Livingstone.

Illsley, R. (2002) 'A city's schools: from equality of input to inequality of output', *Oxford Review of Education*, vol 28, no 4, pp 427–45.

Institute of Almoners (1946), *Memorandum on the care of the chronic sick*, May, London: Institute of Almoners.

International Bank for Reconstruction and Development (1994) *Averting the old age crisis: Policies to protect the old and promote growth*, New York, NY: Oxford University Press.

Jefferys, M. (1997) 'Social medicine and medical sociology 1950–1970s: the testimony of a partisan participant', in D. Porter (ed) *Social medicine and medical sociology in the twentieth century*, Amsterdam, GA: Rodophi.

Jenkins, J.R.F. (1956) *British Medical Journal*, Supplement 1, p 352.

Jewkes, J. and S. (1961) *The genesis of the British National Health Service*, Oxford: Basil Blackwell.

Kelly, D. Lowell (1957) *Journal of Medical Education*, Part 2, pp 195-6.

Kelsall, R.K. (1957) *Report on an Inquiry into Applications for Admission to Universities*, London: HMSO.

Kennedy, C. (1957) *Human disease*, Harmondsworth: Penguin.

Kennedy Commission (2001) *Learning from Bristol: The report of the public inquiry into children's heart surgery, 1984-95*, Cm 5207, London: The Stationery Office.

King Edward's Hospital Fund for London and the Voluntary Hospitals Committee for London (1945) *Some aspects of the post-war hospital problems in London and the home counties*, July, London: King Edward's Hospital Fund for London and the Voluntary Hospitals Committee for London.

King, T. (1934) *Mothercraft*, Sydney, Australia: Whitcombe and Tombs.

Klein, R. (1995) *The new politics of the NHS* (3rd edn), London: Longman.

Klein, R. (2001) *The new politics of the NHS*, Harlow: Prentice Hall.

Krugman, P. (2004) 'The health of nations', *The New York Times*, 17 March.

Lafitte, F. (1961) *Queen's Medical Magazine*, Birmingham, November, p 223.

Lampman, R.J. (1959) *Review of Economic Statistics*, vol 41, November, pp 379-92.

Landis, B.Y. (ed) (1955) 'Ethical standards and professional conduct', *Annals of the American Academy of Political and Social Science*, p 297.

Landis, B.Y. (1956) 'Medicine and the drug industry in Germany', *The Lancet*, vol 2, p 290.

Lees, D.S. (1961) *Health through choice*, London: Institute of Economic Affairs.

Lees, D.S. (1965) 'Health through choice', in R. Harris, *Freedom or free-for-all?*, Hobart Papers, vol 3, London: The Institute of Economic Affairs.

Le Grand, J. (2003) *Motivation, agency and public policy: Of knights and knaves, pawns and queens*, Oxford: Oxford University Press.

Lewis-Faning, E. (1938) *Reports on public health and medical subjects*, No 86, London: HMSO.

Levi-Strauss, C. (1969) *The elementary structures of kinship* (ed R. Needham, 1969) London: Eyre & Spottiswoode.

Levy, H. (1944) *National health insurance*, Cambridge: Cambridge University Press.

Life Offices' Association (1957) *The pension problem: A statement of principle and a review of the Labour Party's proposals*, London: Life Offices' Association.

Little, E.M. (1932) *History of the British Medical Association, 1832-1932*, compiled by E.M. Little, London: British Medical Association.

Logan, W.P.D. (1950) *Population Studies*, vol 4, no 2, p 132.

MacLean, B.C. (1960) 'Group health insurance of America', *Health and Welfare Newsletter*, April, p 2.

McGonigle, G.C.M. and Kirby, J. (1936) *Poverty and public health*, London: Gollancz.

Marmot, M.G. and Wilkinson, R.J. (eds) (1999) *Social determinants of health*, Oxford: Oxford University Press.

Marwick, A. (1982) *British society since 1940*, London: Penguin.

Mauss, M. (1954) *The gift*, translated by I. Cunnison with an introduction by E.E. Evans-Pritchard, London: Routledge.

Mead, G.H. (1934) *Mind, self and society*, Chicago, Il: University of Chicago Press.

Mead, M. (1952) in E. Staley (ed) *Creating an industrial civilization*, New York, NY: Harper & Bros.

Means, R., Morbey, H. and Smith, R. (2002) *From community care to market care: The development of welfare services for older people*, Bristol: The Policy Press.

Mencher, S. (1967) *Private practice and the National Health Service*, Occasional Papers on Social Administration, no 24, London: G. Bell & Sons.

Miller, R. (1926) *British Medical Journal*, vol 2, no 2, supplement p 5.

Miller, R. (1934a) *The Lancet*, vol 1, p 1301.

Miller, R. (1934b) *Proceedings of the Royal Society of Medicine*, vol 24, p 959.

Miller, R. (1937) *British Encyclopaedia of Medical Practice*, vol 6, p 234, London [publisher unknown].

Ministry of Health (1904), *Report of the Inter-Departmental Committee on Physical Deterioration*, Cmd 2176, London: HMSO.

Ministry of Health (1924) *Reports on Public Health Medicine*, no 23, London: HMSO.

Ministry of Health (1927) *Reports on Public Health Medicine*, no 44, London: HMSO.

Ministry of Health (1944) *A National Health Service*, Cmd 6502, London: HMSO.

Ministry of Health (1945a) *Hospital survey of the Yorkshire area*, London: HMSO.

Ministry of Health (1945b) *Hospital survey of the South-Western area*, London: HMSO.

Ministry of Health (1945c) *Hospital survey of South Wales and Monmouthshire*, London: HMSO.

Ministry of Health (1954) *Report of the Committee on the Economic and Financial Problems of the Provisions for Old Age*, Cmd 9333, London: HMSO.

Ministry of Health (1957) *Report of the Committee to Consider the Future Number of Medical Practitioners*, London: HMSO.

Ministry of Health (1959) *Final Report of the Committee on the Cost of Prescribing*, London: HMSO.

Ministry of Labour (1966) *Preservation of pension rights*, Report of a Committee of the National Joint Advisory Council, London: HMSO.

Money Chiozza, L.G. (1912) *Insurance versus poverty*, London: Methuen.

Morris, J.N. (1941) *The Lancet*, vol 1, p 51.

Morris, J.N. (1957) *Uses of epidemiology*, Edinburgh/London: E & S Livingstone.

Morris, J.N. (1964) *Uses of epidemiology*, Edinburgh/London: E & S Livingstone.

Morris, J.N., and Heady, J.A. (1955) 'Social and biological factors in infant mortality', *The Lancet*, vol 1, p 554.

Morris, J.N. and Titmuss, R.M. (1942) 'The epidemiology of juvenile rheumatism', *The Lancet*, vol 2, pp 59-73.

Mullan, P. (2000) *The imaginary timebomb: Why an ageing population is not a social problem*, London: Tauris & Co.

Murphy, S. and Egger, M. (2002) 'Studies of the social causes of tuberculosis in Germany before the First World War: extracts from Mosse and Tugendreich's landmark book', *International journal of epidemiology*, vol 31, pp 742-9.

Myrdal, G. (1944) *An American dilemma: The negro problem and modern democracy*, New York, NY: Harper & Bros.

Newman, C. (1957) *The evolution of medical education in the nineteenth century*, London: Oxford University Press.

Newman, G. (1927) *Reports on public health and medical subjects*, No 44, London: HMSO.

Newsholme, A. (1895) *The Lancet*, vol 1, p 592.

Nightingale, F. (1860) *Notes on nursing: What it is and what it is not*, a facsimile of the first edition published, London: D. Appleton & Co.

Nolte, E. and McKee, M. (2003) 'Measuring the health of nations: analysis of mortality amenable to health care', *British Medical Journal*, vol 327, pp 1129-32.

Office of Policy Planning and Research (1965) *The Negro family: The case for national action*, WA: US Department of Labor.

O'Neill, J. (1972) *Sociology as a skin trade: Essays towards a reflexive sociology*, London: Heinemann Educational.

Orshansky, M. (1963) *Social Security Bulletin*, July, Social Security Administration, WA: US Department of Health.

Owen, D.S., Spain, B. and Weaver, N. (1968) *A unified health service*, Oxford: Pergamon.

Paul, B.D. (1955) *Health, culture and community: Case studies of public health reactions to health programs*, New York, NY: Russell Sage Foundation.

Paul, J.R. (1943) *Epidemiology of rheumatic fever: Some of its public health aspects*, NY [publisher unknown].

Péquignot, H. (1954) *Impact of science on society*, vol 5, no 4, p 256.

Pemberton, J. (2003) 'Malnutrition in England', *International Journal of Epidemiology*, vol 32, pp 493-5.

Perry, B. and Roberts, F. (1937) *British Medical Journal*, vol 2, supplement, p 154.

Peterson, O.L., Andrews, L.P., Spain, R.S. and Greenberg, B.G. (1956) *Journal of Medical Education*, vol 31 (12), part 2.

Poinstard, P.J. (1958) *Medical Economics*, 7 July, p 42.

Poynton, F.J. (1938) *Proceedings of the International Congress of Rheuma. Hydrol.*, London, p 174.

Prentice, C.R.M. (1963) 'The land of the million elephants', *The Lancet*, vol 2, p 290.

Prest, A.R. and Adams, A.A. (1954), *Consumers' expenditure in the United Kingdom, 1900-19*, Cambridge: Cambridge University Press.

Pulvertaft, R.J.V. (1952) *The Lancet*, vol 2, p 839.

Rabin, M. (1997) *Psychology and economics*, Berkeley Department of Economics, Working Paper No 97-251, January, Berkeley, CA: University of California (shorter version published in *Journal of Economic Literature*, March 1998, vol 36, pp 11-46).

Ratner, H. (1962) *Medicine*, Santa Barbara, CA: Center for the Study of Democratic Institutions.

Rawls, J. (1973) *A theory of justice*, Oxford: Oxford University Press.

Registrar-General (1919) *Registrar-General's 75th statistical review, England and Wales,* Supplement, Part 3, London: HMSO.

Registrar-General (1936) *Registrar-General's Statistical review, England and Wales,* London: HMSO.

Registrar-General (1952) *Registrar-General quarterly return, England and Wales (December)*, London: HMSO.

Revell, J.R.S, (1964) in J.E. Meade (ed) *Efficiency, equality and the ownership of property*, London: Allen & Unwin.

Roberts, F. (1952) *The cost of health*, London: Turnstile Press.

Roberts, M. (1959) 'Trends in the supply and demand of medical care', Study Paper No 5, Joint Economic Committee, US Congress, Washington, WA: U.S. Public Health Service.

Roberts, M. (1962) 'Current trends in organization of health services', Conference Papers on the Economics of Health and Medical Care, Michigan, MI: University of Michigan.

Romano, J. (1957) *Tomorrow's challenge to the medical* sciences, London: [publisher unknown].

Rozenthal, A.A. in M.K Sanders (ed) *The crisis in American medicine*, New York, NY: Harper & Bros.

Runciman, W.G. (1966) *Relative deprivation and social justice*, London: Routledge.

Salo, M.A. (1982) *Titmuss, Mauritius and the social population policy: A methodological study*, Turku, Finland: Turun Yliopisto.

Sankey Committee (1937) *Report of the Voluntary Hospitals Commission*, London: British Hospitals Association.

Savage, W.G. (1931) *British Medical Journal*, vol 2, supplement, p 37.

Schlesinger, B. (1937) *Recent advances in the study of rheumatism*, London [publisher unknown].

Schlesinger, B. (1938) *The Lancet*, vol 1, pp 593 and 649.

Schultz, T.W. (1963) *The economic value of education*, New York, NY: Columbia University Press.

Seldon, A. (1957) *Pensions in a free society*, London: Institute of Economic Affairs.

Senn, M.J.E. (ed) (1950) *Symposium on the healthy personality*, New York, NY: [publisher unknown].

Seymour, D. (1959) *The Wall Street Journal*, 27 April, p 1.

Shannon, H.A. and Grebenik, E. (1943) *The population of Bristol*, Cambridge: Cambridge University Press.

Sherrington, C. (1955 edn) *Man on his nature*, Harmondsworth, Penguin.

Sigerist, H.E. (1945) *Civilization and disease*, Ithaca, NY: University of Cornell.

Simmons, L.W. and Wolff, H.G. (1954) *Social science in medicine*, New York, NY: Russell Sage Foundation.

Slack, K.M. (1960) *Councils, committees and concern for the old*, Occasional Papers in Social Administration, No 2, London: London School of Economics and Political Science.

Smith, J. (1996) 'The OPCS longitudinal study', *Social Trends*, London: HMSO.

Smith, R. (2003) 'Is the NHS getting better or worse?', *British Medical Journal*, vol 327, pp 1239-41.

Solzhentisyn, A. (1969) *Cancer ward*, vol 2, trans. N. Bethell and D. Burg, London: Bodley Head.

Somers, H.M. and Somers, A.R. (1964) *Doctors, patients and health insurance* [publisher unknown].

Spence, J.P. (1960) *The purpose and practice of medicine*, Oxford: Oxford University Press.

Spens Committee (1946) *Report of the Inter-Departmental Committee on the Remuneration of General Practitioners*, May, Cmd 6810, London: HMSO.

Starr, D. (1998) *Blood: An epic history of medicine and commerce*, New York, NY: Warner Books.

Sutherland Commission (1999) *With respect to old age: long term care – rights and responsibilities*, Report of the Royal Commission on Long Term Care, March, Cm 4192-I, London: The Stationery Office.

Swift, H. (1940) *Journal of the American Medical Association*, vol 115, p 1509.

Tawney, R.H. (1964) *Equality*, London: Allen & Unwin.

Taylor, M.G. (1956) *The administration of health insurance in Canada*, Toronto: Oxford University Press.

Taylor, S. (1954) *Good general practice*, Oxford: Oxford University Press.

Thornton, C.E. (1938) *Report of the Sch. Medical Officer, London County Council*, vol 3, part 2, London [publisher unknown].

Townsend, P. (1964) *The last refuge*, London: Routledge and Kegan Paul.

Townsend, P. and Davidson, N. (1982) *Inequalities in health: The Black Report*, London: Penguin.

Tuckett, D. (1976) *An introduction to medical sociology*, London: Tavistock.

US Public Health Service (1959) *Physicians for a Growing America*, Report of the Surgeon General's Consultant Group on Medical Education, Washington, WA: US Public Health Service.

US Public Health Service (1961) *Chart book on health status and health manpower*, Washington, WA: US Public Health Service.

Wadsworth, M.E.J., Montgomery, S.M. and Bartley, M.J. (1999) 'The persisting effect of unemployment on health and social well-being in men in early working life', *Social Science and Medicine*, vol 48, pp 1491-9.

Wakeley, C. (1957), *The Lancet*, vol 2, p 906.

Watts, G. (2000) 'Exercising his passion', *British Medical Journal*, vol 321, pp 198-9.

Wanlass, D. (2004) *Securing good health for the whole population*, London: The Stationery Office.

Webb, B. and Webb, S. (1910), *The State and the doctor*, London: Longman.

Wilkinson, K.D. (1935) *The Lancet*, vol 2, p 411.

Wilkinson, R.G. (1996) *Unhealthy societies*, London: Routledge.

Willcocks, A.J. (1967) *The creation of the NHS*, London: Routledge.

Wilson, A.T.M. (1950) *Human relations*, vol 3, no 1.

Wykoff, J. and Ling, C. (1926) *American Heart Journal*, vol 1, p 446.

Young, M. (1921) *Journal of Hygiene*, vol 20, p 248, Cambridge.

Young, M. (1925) *The Lancet*, vol 2, p 590.

Young, M. and Willmott, P. (1957) *Family and kinship in East London*, London: Routledge and Kegan Paul.

Zborowski, M. (1952) *Journal of Social Issues*, vol 8, no 4, p 27.

Bibliography of work by Richard Titmuss

This section provides details of Titmuss's work referred to in this volume together with information on his other published work and articles on health and health-related issues.

1936

'The birth rate and insurance', *Post Magazine and Insurance Monitor*, 19 December, p 2393.

1938

Poverty and population, London: Macmillan.

1941

With Titmuss, K.C. *Parents revolt: A study of the declining birth-rate in acquisitive societies*, London: Secker & Warburg.

'The cost of living and dying', *New Statesman and Nation*, 3 April.

'War and the birth rate', *Eugenics Review*, vol 33, no 2, pp 49-50.

1942

'Eugenics and poverty' (with F. Lafitte), *Eugenics Review*, vol 33, no 4, pp 106-12.

'The effect of the war on the birth rate', *Eugenics Review*, vol 34, no 1, pp 9-12.

'Infant and maternal mortality', *Eugenics Review*, vol 34, no 3, pp 85-90.

'The epidemiology of juvenile rheumatism', *The Lancet*, 18 July, pp 59-73.

1943

(a) *Birth, poverty and wealth: A study of infant mortality*, London: Hamish Hamilton Medical Books.

(b) 'Camp followers of war', *The Listener*, 7 October.

'The significance of recent birth-rate figures', *Eugenics Review*, vol 35, no 2, pp 36-8.

'The social environment and eugenics', *Eugenics Review*, vol 36, p 1802.

1944

'The social environment and eugenics', *Eugenics Review*, vol 36, no 2, July, pp 53-8.

'London and New York: on infant mortality', *The Lancet*, 2 December, p 728.

'Fewer children: the population problem', *Current Affairs*, Army Bureau of Current Affairs, 2 December.

'The epidemiology of peptic ulcer: vital statistics' (with J.N. Morris), *The Lancet*, 30 December, pp 841-56.

with Morris, J.N. (1944) 'Health and social change: (1) The recent history of rheumatic heart disease', *The Medical Officer*, 26 August.

1945

'The statistics of parenthood', in J. Marchant (ed) *Rebuilding family life in the post-war world: An enquiry with recommendations*, Oldhams Press.

1946

'Childlessness and the small family: a fertility survey of Luton' (with F. Grundy), *The Lancet*, 9 November, pp 687ff.

1948

'Parenthood and social change', Lloyd Roberts Lecture for 1948, *The Lancet*, 20 November, pp 797-809.

1950

Problems of social policy (Volume One on the Social Services in the series of Civil Histories of the Second World War), London: HMSO.

1951

'The ministry of health', *The Lancet*, 3 March.

1952

'The cost of medical care: American experience and the NHS', *The Lancet*, 22 March, pp 605-6.

'Medicine without ethics', *New Statesman and Nation*, 5 April.

'The hospital and its patients', *The Hospital*, June.

1954
'Some fundamental assumptions', Third International Congress of Gerontology, London; Old Aged in the Modern World, Proceedings of 3rd Congress, International Association of Gerontology, Edinburgh, and E & S Livingstone.

1956
With Abel-Smith, B. *The cost of the National Health Service in England and Wales*, Cambridge: Cambridge University Press.

1957
'Foreword', in J.P. Martin, *Social aspects of prescribing*, London: Routledge & Kegan Paul.

1958
Essays on 'The welfare state', London: Allen & Unwin.

'Introduction', *Cross-national surveys: Report by the International Association of Gerontology*.

1959
'Community care as a challenge', *The Times*, 12 May.

'Health', in M. Ginsberg (ed) *Law and opinion in England in the twentieth century*, London: Stevens & Sons.

1961
With Abel-Smith, B. with Lynes, T. (1961) *Social policies and population growth in Mauritius*, London: Methuen.

'Community care: fact or fiction?' *The Spectator*, 17 March.

'Historical sedatives', *New Society*, 16 June.

1962
(a) 'Foreword', in M. Young and P. Willmott (eds) *Family and kinship in East London*, Harmondsworth: Penguin.

(b) *Income distribution and social change: A study in criticism*, London: Allen & Unwin.

'Pensioners of privilege', *New Society*, 14 September.

'Planning and population', *New Society*, 8 November.

'The National Health Service in England', in S.N. Eisenstadt (ed) *Comparative social problems*, New York, NY: The Free Press.

1963

(a) 'What British doctors really think about socialized medicine', *Harper's Magazine*, vol 226, February, pp 16-22.

(b) *Essays on 'The welfare state'* (2nd edn), London: Allen & Unwin.

1964

'Planning for ageing: the division of labour in the health and wealth services', *Proceedings of the National Old People's Welfare Conference*, April.

'The future of the family doctor', *New Society*, 30 July, pp 11-3.

'Social and ethnic aspects of therapeutics', in P. Talalay (ed) *Drugs in our society*, Baltimore, MD: Johns Hopkins Press.

'The hospital and its patients', in J. Farndale (ed) *Trends in the Mental Health Services*, Oxford: Pergamon Press.

1965

'The role of the family doctor today in the context of British social services', *The Lancet*, 2 January, pp 1-4.

'Poverty vs inequality: diagnosis', *The Nation*, 8 February, pp 130-3.

'Community care of the mentally ill: some British observations', *Canada's Mental Health*, Supplement, 49, November-December, pp 1-8.

1966

'Forenote', in M. King (ed) *Medical care in developing countries: A symposium from Makerere* (experimental edition assisted by UNICEF), New York, NY: UNICEF.

1968

(a) 'Goals of today's welfare state', in J.A. Kahl (ed) *Comparative perspective on stratification: Mexico, Great Britain, Japan*, Boston, MA: Little, Brown & Co.

(b) 'Ethics and economics of medical care', in *Commitment to welfare*, London: Allen & Unwin.

(c) *Commitment to welfare*, London/New York, NY: Allen & Unwin/ Pantheon.

1969

'The culture of medical care and consumer behaviour', in F.N.L. Poynter (ed) *Medicine and culture, WI*, pp 129-35.

1970

The gift relationship, London: Allen & Unwin [reissued with new chapters by LSE Books, Oakley and Ashton, 1997].

Published posthumously

1974

with Abel-Smith, B. and Titmuss, K.C. (eds) *Social policy: An introduction*, London, New York, NY: Allen & Unwin/Pantheon.

1976

Commitment to welfare (2nd edn with a new introduction by B. Abel-Smith), London: Allen & Unwin.

The irresponsible society (3rd edn with a new introduction by B. Abel-Smith), London: Allen & Unwin.

1987

Abel-Smith, B. and Titmuss, K.C. (eds) (1987) *The philosophy of welfare* (with an introduction by S.M. Miller), London: Allen & Unwin.

1997

Oakley, A. and Ashton, J. (eds) (1977) *The gift relationship: From human blood to social policy by Richard M. Titmuss, original edition with new chapters*, London: LSE Books.

2002

Palgrave Macmillan Archive edition of the writings on social policy and welfare of Richard M. Titmuss, seven volumes, Houndsmill, Basingstoke: Palgrave Macmillan.

Richard Titmuss: further reading

Abel-Smith, B. (1973) 'Richard Morris Titmuss', *Journal of Social Policy*, vol 2, no 3, July.

Deacon, A. (1993) 'Richard Titmuss 20 years on', *Journal of Social Policy*, April, vol 22, no 2, pp 235-42.

Donnison, D. (1973) 'Richard Titmuss', *New Society*, 12 April.

Fontaine, P. (2002) 'Blood, politics and social science: Richard Titmuss and the Institute of Economic Affairs, 1957-73', *Isis* (History of Science Society, Washington DC), vol 93, no 2.

Gowing, M. (1975) 'Richard Morris Titmuss, 1907-73', *Proceedings of the British Academy*, vol 61.

Marshall, T.H. (1973) 'Richard Titmuss – an appreciation', *British Journal of Sociology*, vol 24, no 2.

Murphy, S. (1999) 'The early days of the MRC Social Medicine Research Unit', *Social History of Medicine*, vol 12, no 3, pp 389-406.

Oakley, A. (1991) 'Eugenics, social medicine and the career of Richard Titmuss in Britain 1935-50', *British Journal of Sociology*, vol 42, no 2, pp 165-94.

Oakley, A. (1996) *Man and wife: Richard and Kay Titmuss – My parents' early years*, London: HarperCollins.

Oakley, A. (1997) 'Making medicine social: the case of two dogs with bent legs'. in D Porter (ed) *Social medicine and medical sociology in the twentieth century*, Amsterdam: Rodopi.

Reisman, D.A. (1977) *Richard Titmuss: Welfare and society*, with preface by R.A. Pinker, London: Heineman (2nd edn, 2001), Basingstoke: Palgrave Macmillan.

Rose, H. (1981) 'Rereading Titmuss: the sexual division of welfare', *Journal of Social Policy*, vol 10, no 4, pp 477-502.

Vaizey, J. (1983) *In breach of promise: Gaitskell, Macleod, Titmuss, Crossland, Boyle: Five men who shaped a generation*, London: Weidenfeld & Nicolson.

Watson, D. (1980) 'Richard Titmuss: social policy and social life', in N. Timms (ed) *Social welfare: Why and how?*, London: Routledge.

Welshman, J. (1998) 'Evacuation and social policy during the Second World War: myth and reality', *Twentieth Century British History*, vol 9, no 1, pp 28-53.

Wilding, D. (1976) 'Richard Titmuss and social welfare', *Social and Economic Administration*, vol 10, no 3.

Index

A

Abel-Smith, Brian 3-4, 90, 168, 183
Acheson report (1998) 23
ageing population
  costs in US health care 113
  planning services for 120-1, 151-60
  see also pensions
agency of poor 161-2
altruism 118
  blood donation 175-82
  and respect for client 162-3
  ultimatum game 163
American Civil War 55
American health care system 62, 100, 107-14
  blood donation 177-9
  costs 107-8, 111-12, 112-13
  critique of 168-9
  customer satisfaction 109, 119
  general practice 128-9
  health-consciousness 85-6, 130
  imperfections 110-13
  maldistribution of facilities 108-9
American Hospital Association 104
American Medical Association 85, 103, 109
area differences *see* regional differences
Arrow, K.J. 173
artisan theory of disease 35-6, 41
Attlee government 60
audit evaluation 140-1
autocratic behaviour 138

B

Bach, F. 52
'bad risks' 169-70
Bagehot, Walter 76
Baird, Dugald 202
Barker, D.J.P. 22
bed numbers
  in American hospitals 108
  in pre-war hospitals 68
Bell, Daniel 168
Berkeley, C. 35
Bevan, Aneurin 61, 74
bioterrorism threat 60
birth rate *see* fertility rate
blood donation 175-82
  increasing demand for blood 176, 181
  supply factors 176-7, 181-2
Bloom, S. 119
Boer War 55, 59, 65, 76
British Medical Association 79, 80, 81, 97, 104
British Medical Association Committee 35

C

certification of illness 187
charlatanism 109
Chesterton, G.K. 152
children
  juvenile rheumatism 22-4, 33-41, 44-5, 52-3, 54
  see also infant mortality
Churchill, Edward 133, 135-6
Clark-Kennedy, A.E. 83, 130, 139
class *see* social class
climate and rheumatic heart disease 38, 40, 41
Coburn, A.F. 39
cohort effect 20

Also available from The Policy Press

Welfare and wellbeing
Richard Titmuss's contribution to social policy
Edited by Pete Alcock, Howard Glennerster, Ann Oakley and Adrian Sinfield

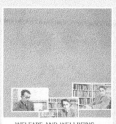

Despite its continuing relevance to current social policy issues both in the UK and internationally, much of Titmuss's work is now out of print. This book brings together a selection of his most important writings on a range of key social policy issues, together with commentary on these from contemporary experts in the field.

The book should be read by undergraduate and postgraduate students in social policy and sociology, for many of whom Titmuss remains compulsory reading. It will be of interest to academics and other policy analysts as well as students and academics in political science and social work.

Paperback ISBN 1 86134 299 3 • £18.99 • (US$29.95) • 240 x 172mm • 256 pages • October 2001

To order further copies of this publication or any other Policy Press titles please contact:

In the UK and Europe:
Marston Book Services, PO Box 269 Abingdon, Oxon, OX14 4YN, UK
Tel: +44 (0)1235 465500
Fax: +44 (0)1235 465556,
Email: direct.orders@marston.co.uk

In the USA and Canada:
ISBS, 920 NE 58th Avenue, Suite 300, Portland, OR 97213-3786, USA
Tel: +1 800 944 6190 (toll free)
Fax: +1 503 280 8832,
Email: info@isbs.com

In Australia and New Zealand:
DA Information Services, 648 Whitehorse Road Mitcham, Victoria 3132, Australia
Tel: +61 (3) 9210 7777
Fax: +61 (3) 9210 7788,
E-mail: service@dadirect.com.au

Further information about all of our titles can be found on our website

www.policypress.org.uk

Printed and bound by CPI Group (UK) Ltd, Croydon, CR0 4YY

09/06/2025

14685900-0002